Solvent-Responsive Shape Memory Polymers for Biomedical Applications

This book explains the intricacies of one-way shape memory polymers (SMPs), with a particular emphasis on solvent-responsive SMPs focusing on fundamental pathways and key principles crucial to the development of these materials. The subsequent section homes in on the specific realm of solvent-responsive SMPs, highlighting the potential advantages these polymers offer and critical evaluation of existing shortcomings and research gaps. It further explains how solvent-responsive SMPs aim to address challenges and advancements within the biomedical industry.

Features:

- Delve into the latest developments and research findings on solvent-responsive shape memory polymers.
- Explore practical and real-world applications of solvent-responsive shape memory polymers in the biomedical domain.
- Provide an understanding of these polymers from molecular to macroscopic levels.
- Explore the underlying physics, chemistry, and thermodynamics that govern the mechanism of solvent-driven shape change in these polymers.
- Review innovations in the design of solvent-responsive shape memory polymers and their applications across a variety of industrial fields.
- Examine how solvent-responsive shape memory polymers can be integrated and applied across different scientific disciplines.

This book is aimed at graduate students and researchers in polymer engineering, materials science, and bioengineering.

Solvent-Responsive Shape Memory Polymers for Biomedical Applications

Sayan Basak and Abhijit Bandyopadhyay

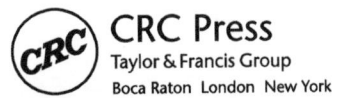

CRC Press
Taylor & Francis Group
Boca Raton London New York

CRC Press is an imprint of the
Taylor & Francis Group, an **Informa** business

CRC Press
Boca Raton and London
First edition published 2025
by CRC Press
2385 NW Executive Center Drive, Suite 320, Boca Raton FL 33431

and by CRC Press
4 Park Square, Milton Park, Abingdon, Oxon, OX14 4RN

CRC Press is an imprint of Taylor & Francis Group, LLC
© 2025 Sayan Basak and Abhijit Bandyopadhyay

ISBN: 9781032862453 (hbk)
ISBN: 9781032974552 (pbk)
ISBN: 9781003593805 (ebk)

DOI: 10.1201/9781003593805

Typeset in Times
by codeMantra

To Ma, Baba and Dida
To Ma, Baba, Anusua and Ahona
To the Department of Polymer Science and Technology, University
  of Calcutta

Contents

Preface

As we began exploring the world of smart polymers, our initial curiosity centered on their reactions to heat and microwave radiation. However, this early interest soon expanded, leading us into a fascinating array of discoveries within this field.

One particular aspect that captivated our attention was shape memory polymers that respond to solvents. These materials possess the remarkable ability to alter their shape upon contact with specific liquids and then revert to their original form. This intriguing property sparked our enthusiasm and drove us to delve deeper into our research.

Reflecting on our journey, we recall countless hours spent in the lab, tackling challenges and celebrating breakthroughs. Each small discovery contributed to our growing understanding of smart polymers, shaping the course of our research.

With this brief, we aim not only to share our findings but also to invite others into the captivating world of shape memory polymers. Our goal is to highlight the extraordinary potential of these materials and inspire further exploration and innovation.

We extend our heartfelt gratitude to everyone who has supported us along the way—our mentors, colleagues, and supporters. Their guidance and encouragement have been invaluable.

To you, the reader, thank you for joining us on this journey. We hope this review ignites a passion for smart polymers and encourages continued research and innovation in this exciting field.

Acknowledgments

We would like to acknowledge Dr. Srijoni Sengupta, Ms. Poulami Dasgupta, and Dr. Tamalika Das for introducing the concept of stimuli-responsive polymers in our laboratory. Working with these materials has been an amazing journey since then. Their insights and guidance have been instrumental in shaping our research and understanding of smart polymers.

We also extend our gratitude to the reviewers who meticulously reviewed our work and provided invaluable suggestions. Their thorough feedback has significantly enhanced the quality and informativeness of this book, making it more beneficial for our readers.

Finally, we express our heartfelt thanks to you, the readers. We hope this book serves as a valuable resource in your scientific endeavors and inspires further exploration and innovation in the fascinating field of smart polymers.

Dr. Sayan Basak
Prof. Abhijit Bandyopadhyay
Kolkata

Author Biography

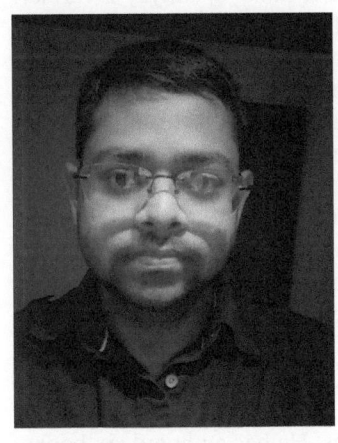

Dr. Sayan Basak completed his B.Tech. in Polymer Science and Technology at the University of Calcutta, India, and earned his Ph.D. from the University of Akron, USA, specializing in smart polymers. His research focused on shape memory and functional polymers, aligning with his undergraduate studies. Post his Ph.D., he worked with Biocon India, where he worked with living ionic polymerization. He is currently an ETH domain research fellow at the Swiss Federal Laboratories for Materials Science and Technology (Empa, *Eidgenössische Materialprüfungs- und Forschungsanstalt*), Switzerland, focusing on catalytic polymerization and chemical reactor engineering. Dr. Basak remains a prominent collaborator of the Bandyopadhyay Lab at the University of Calcutta. He collaborates in the domains of polymer chemistry, polymer physics, and polymer structure-property relationships.

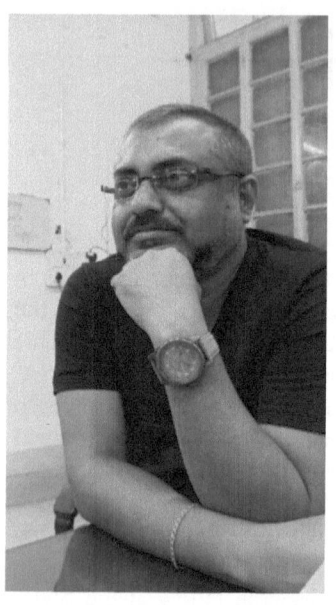

Prof. Dr. Abhijit Bandyopadhyay is currently Full Professor in the Department of Polymer Science & Technology at the University of Calcutta and a member of the Senate of the University. Additionally, he is also acting as the Technical Director of South Asia Rubber and Polymers Park, West Bengal. Dr. Bandyopadhyay is former Head of the Department and the member of the Syndicate of this University. He is a National Scholar and has received Young Scientist Award in 2005 from Material Research Society of India and Kolkata Chapter and Career Award for Young Teachers in 2010 from Govt. of India for his contribution in teaching and research in various domains of polymer and rubber science and technology. He has published more than 110 research papers in reputed international journals, authored 5 books, filed 2 Indian patents, and delivered several Plenary, Keynote, and Invited lectures in International and National conferences and Faculty Development Programs. He has authored six books so far. He has also done both Government- and Industry-sponsored research projects and offered industrial consultancies regarding development of several products. He has supervised 12 research students so far for obtaining their Doctorate degree and 10 more are currently doing their research under his supervision. He is the life member of Society of Polymer Science (SPS) and Indian Rubber Institute (IRI) and Associate Member of Indian Institute of Chemical Engineers (IICHE). He is also connected to All India Rubber Industries Association, Eastern Region (AIRIA, ER) and Indian Plastics Institute (IPI). His research interests include polymer blends and composites, polymer nanocomposites, hyperbranched polymers, and polymer 3D printing.

Introduction to Shape Memory Polymers

1

Evolution, Growth, and Market Size

1.1 VERSATILITY AND TRIGGER MECHANISMS

Shape memory polymers (SMPs) constitute a fascinating category of intelligent materials renowned for their ability to retain their original configuration even after undergoing significant deformation—a phenomenon aptly termed the shape memory effect (SME) [1]. What sets SMPs apart is their autonomous capacity to revert to their primary shape without requiring external forces to facilitate the process.

One of the most intriguing aspects of SMPs is their versatility in transitioning between one or more temporary shapes and subsequently returning to their original form when triggered by specific physical stimuli [1]. These stimuli can range from conventional factors like heat to more innovative triggers such as electric or magnetic fields, water, light, or even physiological conditions like pH, body temperature, and ion concentration. Over the years, the realm of SMPs has witnessed a proliferation of diverse materials boasting desirable properties [2,3,4]. These properties include but are not limited to multi-SMEs, ease of processing, and remarkable deformability.

DOI: 10.1201/9781003593805-1

1

Such advancements have significantly expanded the horizons of SMP applications across various domains.

In sensor technology, for instance, SMPs have found remarkable utility owing to their unique responsiveness to external stimuli [5]. They are also making significant inroads into the realm of smart textiles, where their shape-changing abilities offer novel functionalities and enhanced comfort [6]. Moreover, aerospace components are benefiting from the lightweight yet durable nature of SMPs, contributing to advancements in aerospace engineering [7].

Furthermore, the integration of SMPs into robotics has unlocked new possibilities in the development of adaptive and shape-changing robotic systems [8]. In the biomedical field, SMPs hold immense promise for applications ranging from minimally invasive surgical tools to controlled drug delivery systems (Figure1.1) [9].

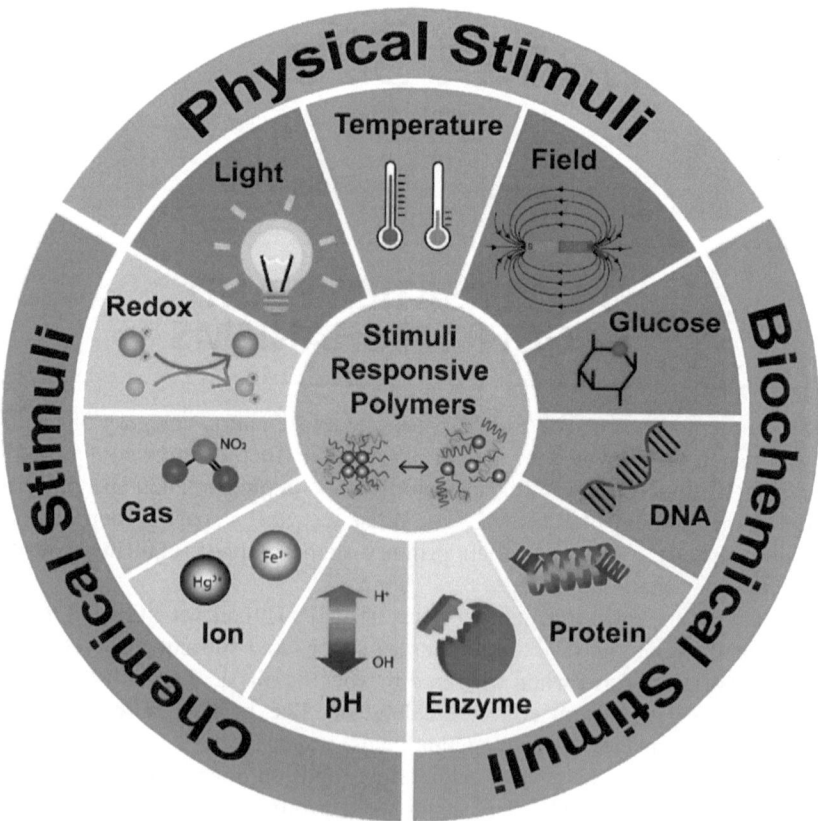

FIGURE 1.1 Physical, chemical, and biochemical responsiveness of stimuli-responsive and shape memory polymers. Reproduced with permission [10], copyright 2020, American Chemical Society.

Usually, SMPs can be categorized using different methods [11]. Nonetheless, a widely used classification approach for these polymers is based on their shape memory characteristics, which include the one-way shape memory effect (1W-SME), the two-way reversible shape memory effect (2W-SME), and the multiple-shape memory effect (MSME) (Figure 1.2) [11–13].

The genesis of SMPs, as elucidated in references [11] and [13], traces back to the exploration of the "one-way shape memory effect." This phenomenon, initially investigated in the mid-20th century, involves the controlled deformation of polymer objects at elevated temperatures, resulting in the elastic stretching of polymer chains. Upon cooling, the material is fixed into a temporary shape, immobilizing the deformed chains, and the original shape can be restored by reheating the material, allowing the polymer chains to revert to their initial configuration.

1.2 HISTORICAL DEVELOPMENT OF SMPS

Historically, the earliest documented reference to shape memory can be found in a 1941 patent, where it was termed "elastic memory," as noted by Liu et al. [13]. Concurrently, terms such as "plastic memory" and "elastic-plastic behavior" were also mentioned in the literature from the same era. Despite the conceptual understanding of plastic memory within the polymer field by the 1960s, practical applications of SMPs were largely confined to commonplace materials like heat shrink tubing, films, and novelties such as polystyrene Shrinky Dinks, as highlighted in reference [5].

However, during this period of exploration, as referenced in [13], more robust applications began to emerge, including the investigation of SMPs for use in space-deployable structures. This exemplifies the gradual expansion of the understanding and application of SMPs beyond traditional uses, paving the way for their eventual integration into diverse industries and cutting-edge technologies.

The emergence of SMPs as a distinct and specialized category of materials during the 1980s marked a significant milestone in the evolution of polymer science and engineering [13]. This pivotal development can be attributed to a confluence of factors that collectively propelled the recognition and exploration of these unique materials. One contributing factor to the delineation of SMPs as a distinct category was the growing interest and research focus on shape memory metals during the same period [13]. The study of shape memory alloys, particularly their remarkable ability to recover their original shape upon heating after deformation, provided

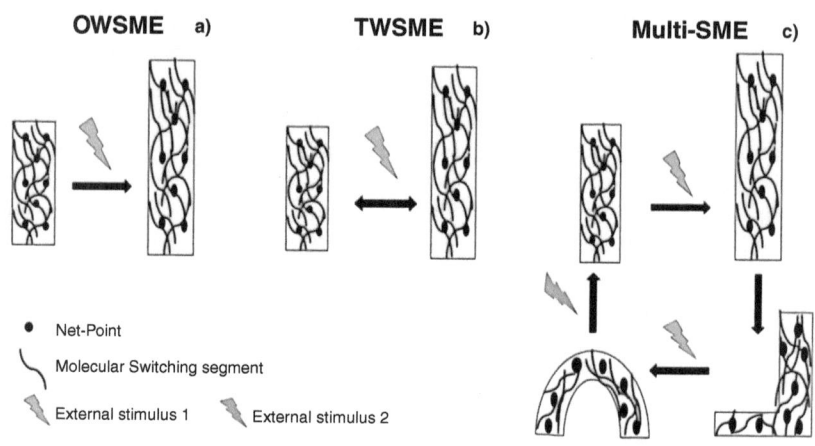

FIGURE 1.2 Illustration representing the one-way shape memory effect (1W-SME), two-way reversible shape memory effect (2W-SME), and multiple-SME (MSME) in shape memory polymers. Reproduced with permission from [12], copyright reserved MDPI 2020.

inspiration and impetus for investigating similar properties in polymeric materials.

Furthermore, the 1980s witnessed a proliferation of diverse polymers capable of exhibiting the one-way SME, coupled with the ability to tailor their structure–property relationships [13]. This increased availability of polymers with customizable properties provided researchers with a rich palette of materials to explore, laying the groundwork for the development of SMPs with tailored functionalities and applications.

Moreover, the burgeoning utility of SMPs in high-value applications, notably within the medical device sector, further underscored the significance of these materials [13]. Their unique combination of mechanical properties, biocompatibility, and shape memory behavior positioned them as promising candidates for a wide range of medical applications, from minimally invasive surgical tools to drug delivery systems.

As the field of polymer science and engineering continued to advance, the domain of SMPs expanded rapidly. Researchers delved into exploring novel chemical compositions, innovative processing techniques, and advanced characterization methods to further enhance the performance and versatility of these materials.

For those interested in delving deeper into the diverse landscape of SMPs, comprehensive reviews within the field serve as invaluable resources

[11]. These reviews offer a comprehensive exploration of various SMPs, covering their synthesis, characterization, properties, and applications, thereby providing a comprehensive understanding of this dynamic and evolving field.

1.3 MARKET GROWTH AND FUTURE PROSPECTS

The global SMP market, as indicated by an extensive study conducted by Future Market Insights, stands on the cusp of remarkable growth in the approaching decade. This in-depth analysis presents a compelling projection, forecasting a notable compound annual growth rate (CAGR) of 26.9% within the timeframe spanning from 2022 to 2032 [4]. As of the base year, 2022, the worldwide SMP market has already exhibited substantial progress, boasting a preliminary valuation estimated at US$ 450.4 million. The growth trajectory foreseen for this market is founded upon a convergence of factors that accentuate the escalating significance and the diverse array of applications associated with SMPs across a broad spectrum of industries. Central to the allure of this market lies the extraordinary property inherent in SMPs, whereby they have the capacity to "remember" their original configuration and revert to it when exposed to specific stimuli, including heat, light, or mechanical force. This singular attribute bestows upon them remarkable versatility and situates them as pivotal materials within numerous sectors, encompassing healthcare, aerospace, automotive, and consumer electronics [5].

The projected market valuation of US$3.5 billion by 2032, as outlined in reference [5], serves as a reinforcement to the surging demand and expansive opportunities within the realm of SMPs. Across diverse sectors, these innovative materials are catalyzing transformative advancements and reshaping the landscape of numerous industries.

In the healthcare sector, SMPs, referenced in [5], are rapidly gaining prominence as indispensable components in cutting-edge medical applications. They are revolutionizing the development of minimally invasive surgical tools, advanced drug delivery systems, and pioneering tissue engineering methodologies. This not only enhances patient outcomes but also underscores the pivotal role of SMPs in driving progress within medical technology. Simultaneously, the automotive and aerospace industries, highlighted in [5], are embracing the potential of SMPs with unwavering enthusiasm. These materials are being integrated into a myriad of applications, including lightweight structural components aimed at boosting fuel efficiency, energy-efficient materials, and responsive surfaces tailored to adapt to dynamic environmental conditions. Such advancements not only improve performance but also contribute to sustainability efforts by reducing fuel consumption and emissions.

Moreover, within the realm of consumer electronics, as referenced in [5], SMPs are playing a transformative role in revolutionizing the design and functionality of electronic devices. Their incorporation into critical components, such as those found in smartphones, significantly enhances user experiences and ensures the enduring durability of electronic products.

In the marked by heightened environmental consciousness, as noted in [4], SMPs offer a compelling solution aligned with sustainability initiatives. Their inherent versatility and eco-friendly attributes present opportunities for the conscientious facilitation of eco-friendly manufacturing processes and the creation of recyclable materials. This resonance with the burgeoning demand for sustainable solutions underscores the enduring relevance and potential of SMPs in addressing global challenges while driving economic growth.

Nevertheless, the anticipated market valuation and burgeoning demand for SMPs underscore their transformative impact across industries, from healthcare to automotive, aerospace, and consumer electronics. As innovation continues to drive progress, SMPs stand poised to play a pivotal role in shaping the future of materials science and engineering. The dynamic and evolving landscape of materials science, characterized by ongoing research and development endeavors, plays an instrumental role in catalyzing the expansion of the SMP market. The pursuit of innovation continues to yield discoveries of novel applications and refinements of existing formulations, thereby propelling market growth and diversification [6].

The projected CAGR of 26.9% forecasted for the global SMP market from 2022 to 2032, along with the anticipated market value reaching US$3.5 billion by 2032, highlights the remarkable growth prospects inherent in this industry. This trajectory of expansion is not mere speculation; rather, it is bolstered by concrete factors, including the pioneering applications emerging in sectors such as healthcare, automotive, aerospace, and consumer electronics [10].

In healthcare, for instance, SMPs are revolutionizing medical devices and implants, offering innovative solutions for personalized medicine, minimally invasive surgeries, and drug delivery systems. Similarly, in the automotive and aerospace sectors, these polymers are enabling the development of lightweight, high-performance materials that enhance fuel efficiency, reduce emissions, and improve overall safety.

Moreover, the growing emphasis on sustainability and advancements in materials science are driving the demand for SMPs. As industries seek greener alternatives and strive for greater efficiency, these versatile materials offer solutions that align with sustainability goals while also delivering superior performance [14,15].

Companies operating within the realm of SMPs find themselves strategically positioned to capitalize on significant opportunities arising from this growth trajectory. By leveraging their expertise in research, development, and manufacturing, these companies can not only meet current market demands but also actively shape the future of the industry. Furthermore, their contributions to advancing the capabilities and applications of SMPs will play a pivotal role in the dynamic evolution of this landscape, fostering innovation and driving progress across various sectors [14–18].

Furthermore, the projected growth and market potential of the global SMP market underscore a compelling narrative of innovation, opportunity, and sustainable development. As industries across the board increasingly recognize the value of these remarkable materials, the stage is set for transformative advancements and collaborative efforts that will shape the future of materials science and engineering [14,15].

1.4 ENVISIONING A BROADER FUTURE

Recent literature [18–20] highlights significant opportunities for further advancements in the field of SMPs. While there is much anticipation for the discovery of novel polymers and their unimaginable applications, there remains a pressing need to enhance specific properties of current SMPs, which restrict their broader application.

Emerging chemical synthesis strategies [21] are paving the way for the development of novel SMP structures. These new systems are expected to deepen our understanding of the structure–property relationships of SMPs [10]. Although our current grasp of the SME mechanism and design principles is robust, especially for simpler one-way dual shape polymers, more complex SME behaviors (e.g., multiple SMEs) demand further investigation. A critical aspect of designing new polymer structures involves tuning the switching temperature (TSW). Many SMP systems were initially inspired by biological applications and thus exhibit low TSWs. However, recent efforts have focused on developing high-temperature SMPs [22], which are crucial for applications requiring excellent thermal stability and mechanical properties, such as aerospace. Future research will likely emphasize tuning the transition temperatures in triple and multiple SMPs, as systems based on broad thermal transitions (e.g., T_g) inherently limit the range of different TSWs.

Systems utilizing two separate phases generally offer a broader range, but only a few examples demonstrate switching temperatures with differences greater than 50 K [22]. TSW has been achieved in several systems by altering the monomers/segments used or the molar mass of the switching segments. Future developments might focus on "post-synthesis" tuning of switching temperatures through additional stress, solvent vapors, or integrating additional switchable units within the SMP itself.

The range of stimuli applicable to the SME is also expected to expand. Currently, external heat (indirect) remains the most commonly applied stimulus. Approaches for internal heating, such as inductive heating [23], resistive heating (e.g., integrated wires, composites with conductive additives) [22,23], infrared irradiation [23], and photothermal heating, are promising. Photo-switchable SMPs could benefit from tuning the wavelength required for switching, either by adjusting the photo-switch or through energy transfer processes (shorter irradiation wavelengths, energy transfer from dye molecules to the switch) and upconversion processes (longer irradiation wavelengths, upconversion on dye/metal complex nanoparticles) [24]. This approach could enable photo-induced switching (NIR region) of SMPs for in vivo applications [2].

Non-thermal stimuli responsiveness makes SMPs ideal candidates for sensor systems. Leveraging the multi-domain morphology of SMPs might lead to polymers triggered by different stimuli (e.g., one domain thermally, another by light). Mechanical forces are also intriguing triggers for SMPs, particularly for structural material applications [25]. Autonomous SMPs (aligned with the definition of self-healing materials) represent another innovative direction. These materials would trigger the SME during use without external intervention (commonly heating). While this goal is still distant, SMPs for bioapplications could serve as preliminary examples, activated by body temperature [22].

New polymer structures aim to enhance shape transformation capabilities. While multiple SMEs have been extensively studied, future developments will focus on improving the fixity and recovery of individual steps. Simple transformations between two different shapes also hold interest. Contrary to the naïve assumption that permanent and temporary shapes can be freely chosen, the permanent shape largely determines the temporary shape. Typically, the polymer sample is heated and strained/coiled to form the temporary shape. Upon reheating, the original shape is almost uniformly recovered through contraction. The pursuit of an "opposite" SMP (heat-induced expansion and contraction upon cooling) would require a novel mechanism, as the current trend is based on molecular mechanisms (e.g., crystallization-induced expansion). The synthesis of novel polymer structures is aimed not only at achieving unprecedented SME properties but also at developing materials suitable for commercial applications. This involves improving properties such as higher fixity and recovery, better stability, higher cycle life, and superior mechanical properties. Mechanical properties are particularly crucial, as many applied polymeric systems are relatively soft, limiting their range of applications. Therefore, materials with better mechanical properties that retain the SMEs are highly desirable. A significant challenge is the loss of mechanical properties at the switching temperature (when the T_g or T_m of one phase is reached). Consequently, the desired mechanical properties must be provided by one of the different phases of the SMP.

Additionally, the processability and availability of current SMPs are critical issues for several applications. Many described polymer structures are ideal for scientific laboratories, but their synthesis and fabrication processes are often not feasible for industrial applications. Crosslinking, often achieved through chemical methods, poses a significant challenge for industrial scalability due to limited processability. Efforts will focus on improving the mechanical properties of physically crosslinked materials, which currently lag behind chemically crosslinked counterparts. The potential production volumes of some SMPs, particularly those with complex architectures, are also limited, restricting their application range. Encouragingly, research on commercially available polymers in the context of SMPs is increasing (e.g., Nafion, polyimides, natural rubber). Even these standard materials have demonstrated fascinating SMEs.

Expanding the complexity of shape transformations through polymer structure tuning will eventually reach its limits. However, even simple patterning of polymer samples with active and inactive areas can open new possibilities [26]. Special processing technologies, such as inkjet printing, enable such patterning [27–29]. For instance, inkjet technology has been used to fabricate patterns of SMP polymers on substrates, allowing for complex folding geometries (e.g., folding a cube) [31]. Controlling the spatial distribution of the SMP enables the creation of complex architectures. Additionally, aligning liquid crystals in liquid crystal elastomers (LCEs) through light or surface-guided assembly opens up further possibilities for tuning SME geometry [27–31].

Multifunctionality will be a significant aspect of novel SMPs [22]. This involves materials that possess SME as a central property alongside another independent property (e.g., biocompatibility). Many potential applications require this multifunctionality. The future challenge will be integrating additional properties into SMPs without interfering with each other.

Programming SMPs is another crucial issue [32]. Polymeric materials provide a platform that can be utilized in various ways through programming. Depending on the programming step, different SMEs can be observed. Multiple SMPs are particularly interesting in this context. Initial investigations have shown that these polymers can be programmed in a single-step procedure, eliminating the need for tedious multi-step programming [22]. This simplification makes these complex SMPs more practical for potential applications.

Looking forward, additional applications of SMPs are anticipated. Currently, three major trends are emerging. Biomedical applications of SMPs are expected to increase due to their excellent properties and the commercial availability of suitable polymers. This field has been a major driving force in the past and will continue to drive future developments. The tunability, soft material nature, switching at body temperature, biocompatibility, and biodegradability of SMPs make them superior to other shape memory materials, such as shape memory alloys. Promising areas include self-deployable stents and minimally invasive surgery.

Another growing field is shape memory fibers for textiles [33]. Various materials (e.g., shape memory polyurethanes) are commercially available for fabricating these fibers. The SME provides functionality for textiles, such as size and shape adjustment, leading to personalized garments. Applications in aerospace are also nearing technical readiness. SMPs will find more commercial applications in consumer goods (e.g., the enfolding chair, reshapeable handles of forks). The materials are ready, awaiting inventive engineers to harness their potential. Other potential applications will also flourish as the material base broadens and more SMPs reach maturity.

Given the wide range of explored applications, predicting entirely unprecedented applications of SMPs is challenging. One potential area is energy storage, particularly for electrochemical energy storage devices (e.g., redox flow batteries). SMPs, although not yet optimized for this purpose, are not far behind classical mechanical systems. While lithium-ion batteries outperform polymers in terms of energy density, the cost and other factors make SMPs a promising alternative.

In the context of this comprehensive book, our primary focus shall be directed toward the examination of one-way SMPs. These specialized materials possess the remarkable capability to revert to their original, or "remembered," configuration when exposed to specific stimuli, including but not limited to changes in temperature, exposure to light, interaction with solvents, or the influence of magnetic fields. Among these, one-way SMPs have garnered particular attention for their capacity to undergo a unidirectional shape recovery process, conferring unique advantages and applications in various scientific and engineering domains. Our forthcoming discussion will center around elucidating the foundational pathways and essential principles integral to the development of stimuli-responsive SMPs. This structured framework is indispensable for comprehending how diverse stimuli can activate the SME within polymer matrices, consequently engendering their distinct ability to exhibit controlled shape transformations and reversibility.

The subsequent section of our book will outline the general pathway for developing stimuli-responsive SMPs, serving as a foundational framework for understanding how different types of stimuli can activate the SME in polymers, ultimately leading to their remarkable ability to exhibit shape transformations and reversibility.

Moreover, we will delve into the realm of solvent-responsive SMPs, shedding light on their significance in the scientific literature. While highlighting their potential advantages, we will also discuss the existing shortcomings and gaps in this area of research. This critical evaluation will pave the way for understanding how solvent-responsive SMPs are striving to bridge these gaps and revolutionize the biomedical industry.

In summary, this concise brief will offer a comprehensive exploration of developmental strategies of one-way SMPs, their development pathways, and their transformative impact on various industries, with a particular focus on the promising domain of solvent-responsive SMPs in biomedical applications.

REFERENCES

1. Lendlein, A., & Kelch, S. (2002). Shape-memory polymers. *Angewandte Chemie International Edition, 41*(12), 2034–2057.
2. Sun, L., & Huang, W. M. (2010). Mechanisms of the multi-shape memory effect and temperature memory effect in shape memory polymers. *Soft Matter, 6*(18), 4403–4406.
3. Melly, S. K., Liu, L., Liu, Y., & Leng, J. (2020). Active composites based on shape memory polymers: Overview, fabrication methods, applications, and future prospects. *Journal of Materials Science, 55*(25), 10975–11051.
4. Chen, Y. C., & Lagoudas, D. C. (2008). A constitutive theory for shape memory polymers. Part I: Large deformations. *Journal of the Mechanics and Physics of Solids, 56*(5), 1752–1765.
5. Kunzelman, J., Chung, T., Mather, P. T., & Weder, C. (2008). Shape memory polymers with built-in threshold temperature sensors. *Journal of Materials Chemistry, 18*(10), 1082–1086.
6. Thakur, S. (2017). Shape memory polymers for smart textile applications. Bipin Kumar (Ed.), In *Textiles for advanced applications* (pp. 323–336), Hong Kong Polytechnic University, China: intechopen.
7. Liu, Y., Du, H., Liu, L., & Leng, J. (2014). Shape memory polymers and their composites in aerospace applications: A review. *Smart Materials and Structures, 23*(2), 023001.

8. Lendlein, A. (2018). Fabrication of reprogrammable shape-memory polymer actuators for robotics. *Science Robotics, 3*(18), eaat9090.
9. Lendlein, A., Behl, M., Hiebl, B., & Wischke, C. (2010). Shape-memory polymers as a technology platform for biomedical applications. *Expert review of Medical Devices, 7*(3), 357–379.
10. Sun, X., Agate, S., Salem, K. S., Lucia, L., & Pal, L. (2020). Hydrogel-based sensor networks: Compositions, properties, and applications—a review. *ACS Applied Bio Materials, 4*(1), 140–162.
11. Nam, S., & Pei, E. (2019). A taxonomy of shape-changing behavior for 4D printed parts using shape-memory polymers. *Progress in Additive Manufacturing, 4*, 167–184.
12. Scalet, G. (2020, February). Two-way and multiple-way shape memory polymers for soft robotics: An overview. *Actuators, 9*(1), 10. MDPI.
13. Basak, S., Dasgupta, P., & Bandyopadhyay, A. (2023). One-way shape memory polyesters-evolution, growth, developments, and current trends. *Polymer-Plastics Technology and Materials, 62*(17), 2286–2317.
14. Basak, S., Angel, J. C. M., & Cavicchi, K. A. (2023). Thermal annealing of high cis-1, 4-polybutadiene/octadecyl acrylate blends as a one-step process for fabricating shape memory polymers. *ACS Applied Polymer Materials, 5*(7), 4738–4752.
15. Basak, S., & Cavicchi, K. A. (2023). Structure–property relationships of shape memory, semicrystalline polymers fabricated by in situ polymerization and crosslinking of octadecyl acrylate/polybutadiene blends. *Macromolecular Rapid Communications, 44*(1), 2200404.
16. Olukman Şahin, M., & Demirbilek Bucak, C. (2023). Hydrophobically associated poly (acrylamide/octadecyl acrylate)-carboxymethyl cellulose hydrogels: Synthesis, characterization, and shape memory ability. *Journal of Polymers and the Environment, 31*(8), 3650–3663.
17. Abdullah, T., & Okay, O. (2023). 4D printing of body temperature-responsive hydrogels based on poly (acrylic acid) with shape-memory and self-healing abilities. *ACS Applied Bio Materials, 6*(2), 703–711.
18. Zende, R., Ghase, V., & Jamdar, V. (2023). A review on shape memory polymers. *Polymer-Plastics Technology and Materials, 62*(4), 467–485.
19. Rokaya, D., Skallevold, H. E., Srimaneepong, V., Marya, A., Shah, P. K., Khurshid, Z., ... & Sapkota, J. (2023). Shape memory polymeric materials for biomedical applications: An update. *Journal of Composites Science, 7*(1), 24.
20. Xia, Y., He, Y., Zhang, F., Liu, Y., & Leng, J. (2021). A review of shape memory polymers and composites: Mechanisms, materials, and applications. *Advanced Materials, 33*(6), 2000713.
21. Berg, G. J., McBride, M. K., Wang, C., & Bowman, C. N. (2014). New directions in the chemistry of shape memory polymers. *Polymer, 55*(23), 5849–5872.
22. Hager, M. D., Bode, S., Weber, C., & Schubert, U. S. (2015). Shape memory polymers: Past, present and future developments. *Progress in Polymer Science, 49*, 3–33.
23. Xu, J., & Song, J. (2011). Thermal responsive shape memory polymers for biomedical applications. *Biomed. Eng. Front. Chall*, 125–142.

24. Yoon, J. (2021). Design-to-fabrication with thermo-responsive shape memory polymer applications for building skins. *Architectural Science Review, 64*(1–2), 72–86.

25. Mather, P. T. (2006). *U.S.* Patent *No. 7,151,157.* Washington, DC: U.S. Patent and Trademark Office.

26. Ge, Q., Qi, H. J., & Dunn, M. L. (2013). Active materials by four-dimension printing. *Appl. Phys. Lett.* 103, 131901.

27. De Gans, B. J., Duineveld, P. C., & Schubert, U. S. (2004). Inkjet printing of polymers: State of the art and future developments. *Advanced Materials, 16*(3), 203–213.

28. Tekin, E., Smith, P. J., & Schubert, U. S. (2008). Inkjet printing as a deposition and patterning tool for polymers and inorganic particles. *Soft Matter, 4*(4), 703–713.

29. de Haan, L. T., Schenning, A. P., & Broer, D. J. (2014). Programmed morphing of liquid crystal networks. *Polymer, 55*(23), 5885–5896.

30. Iqbal, D., & Samiullah, M. H. (2013). Photo-responsive shape-memory and shape-changing liquid-crystal polymer networks. *Materials, 6*(1), 116–142.

31. Anthamatten, M., Roddecha, S., & Li, J. (2013). Energy storage capacity of shape-memory polymers. *Macromolecules, 46*(10), 4230–4234.

32. Hu, J., Zhu, Y., Huang, H., & Lu, J. (2012). Recent advances in shape–memory polymers: Structure, mechanism, functionality, modeling and applications. *Progress in Polymer Science, 37*(12), 1720–1763.

33. Wang, L., Zhang, F., Liu, Y., & Leng, J. (2022). Shape memory polymer fibers: Materials, structures, and applications. *Advanced Fiber Materials, 4*(1), 5–23.

General Pathway for Designing (One-Way) Shape Memory Polymers

2

2.1 INTRODUCTION

Generally, shape memory polymers (SMPs) exhibit a dual-phase structure, comprising a stable network phase and a second phase influenced by an external trigger [1]. The stable network phase plays a pivotal role in stabilizing the entire SMP and is responsible for retaining the original shape. The deformation of this phase serves as the driving force behind shape recovery. Achieving this stable phase can involve introducing chemical crosslinks [2], crystalline phases [3], or interpenetrating networks [1,4,5].

Conversely, the second phase serves the purpose of temporarily fixing the temporary shape through mechanisms such as crystallization (where a melting transition triggers shape recovery) [6], a glass transition [7], transitions between different liquid crystalline phases [8], or the reversible formation of covalent or non-covalent bonds (e.g., photodimerization of coumarin [9], Diels–Alder reactions [10], and supramolecular interactions) [11].

DOI: 10.1201/9781003593805-2

Additionally, domains responsive to other stimuli (e.g., redox reactions) that can undergo segmental rearrangement may be employed [12].

The shape memory effect (SME) is not an inherent intrinsic property within polymers; rather, it is a phenomenon that emerges from a complex interplay between the polymer's inherent morphology and specific processing techniques, effectively constituting a functionalization of the polymer. This unique characteristic allows polymers to exhibit remarkable shape memory behavior [12]. Through conventional manufacturing processes such as extrusion or injection molding, the polymer is initially molded into its permanent form, which is often referred to as the initial shape. This permanent shape serves as the polymer's default configuration under typical conditions. Subsequently, in a pivotal phase termed "programming," the polymer sample is deliberately subjected to deformation and temporarily molded into an alternative configuration known as the programmed shape. This temporary shape is temporarily locked or fixed within the polymer's structure, awaiting the right external stimulus to trigger its recovery.

Upon the application of a specific external stimulus, which can vary depending on the particular polymer and its design, the polymer undergoes a transition, reverting to its original, permanent shape. It's important to note that this programming and recovery cycle can be iterated multiple times, enabling the polymer to exhibit various temporary shapes in subsequent cycles.

The realm of shape memory materials has witnessed the exploration of various stimuli to initiate the intriguing process of shape memory activation. Among these stimuli, thermal, light, solvent, and magnetic forces have consistently maintained their status as the preferred methods for triggering shape transitions. In the subsequent sections, we will provide a comprehensive overview of the fundamental design principles that underlie SMPs activated by these four predominant types of stimuli. We will then delve deeper into the realm of solvent-responsive SMPs, shedding light on their recent advancements and emerging trends, particularly within the dynamic landscape of the biomedical industry.

2.2 GENERAL PATHWAY FOR DESIGNING THERMORESPONSIVE (ONE-WAY) SMPS

The key thermal transitions applied to SMPs primarily involve two distinct block or component phases: the melting temperature and the glass transition temperature (as depicted in Figure 2.1). The melting transition is applicable to chemically crosslinked rubbers, semicrystalline polymeric networks, and physically crosslinked polymers. The latter category encompasses (multi)block copolymers featuring a low-melting phase responsible for the shape-changing process and a high-melting phase constituting the permanent network. Similarly, the glass transition can be harnessed in chemically cross-linked thermosets and physically crosslinked thermoplastics [13].

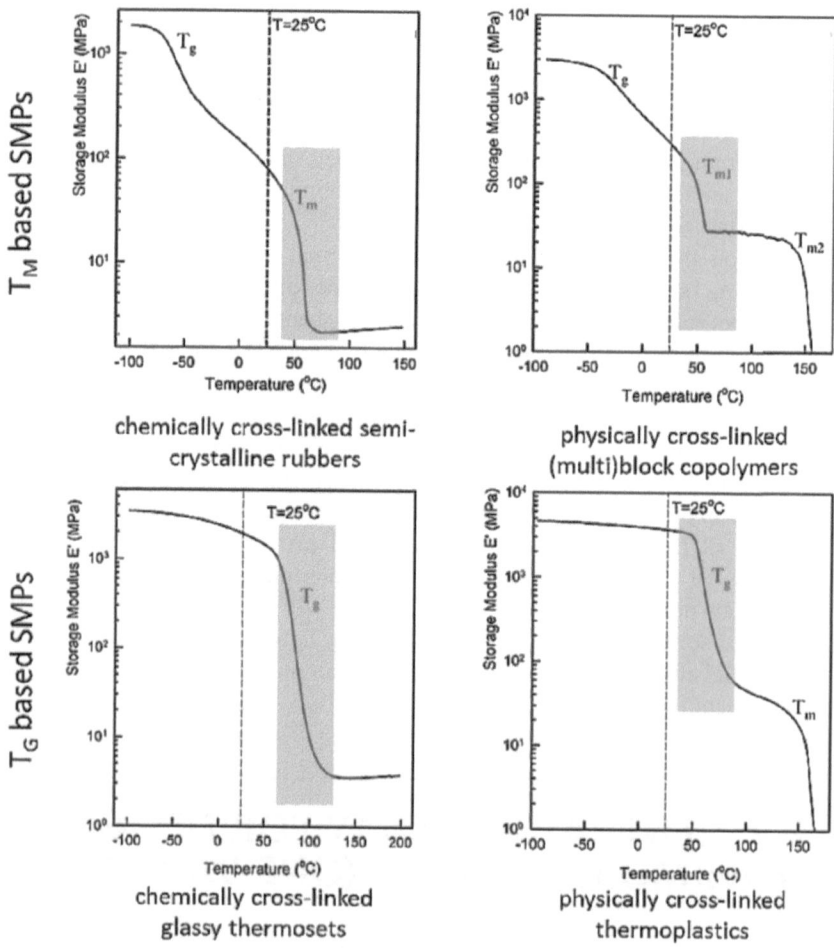

FIGURE 2.1   Melting temperature (T_M) and glass transition temperature (Tg)-based SMPs (the shaded area indicates the switching area of the SMP). Reproduced with permission from [13], copyright reserved Royal Society of Chemistry 2007.

Two crucial parameters are used to quantify the performance of a (one-way) SMP: shape fixity and shape recovery. While shape fixity refers to the ability of the polymer to fix the programmed shape, shape recovery accounts for the extent to which the programmed shape returns to the permanent/original shape when excited with the stimuli [14–16]. A standard cycle (for a thermoresponsive SMP) involves three key phases: shape programming, shape fixation, and shape recovery. In this process, the SMP is subjected to significant deformation, reaching a maximum strain denoted as ε_m, typically achieved at either high or low temperatures. Subsequently, the SMP is cooled down to lower temperatures, typically below the transition temperature of the fixing network, followed by unloading, resulting in a remaining strain denoted as ε_u. The degree of shape fixity is then quantified, as depicted in Figure 2.2.

$$R_f = \frac{\varepsilon_u}{\varepsilon_m} \tag{2.1}$$

The material is heated in the following shape recovery process, and the remaining strain is (ε_h). Shape recovery ratio (R_r) is normally defined as

$$R_r = \frac{\varepsilon_u - \varepsilon_h}{\varepsilon_u} \tag{2.2}$$

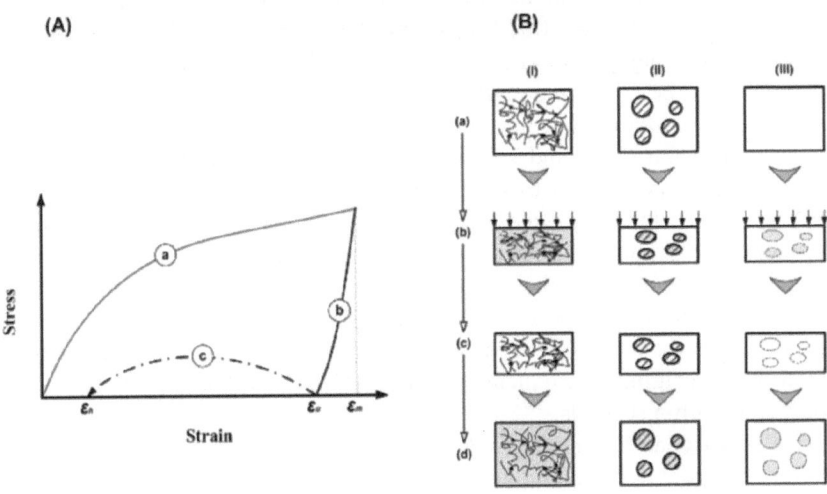

FIGURE 2.2 (a) Illustration of a typical shape memory cycle in heating-responsive shape memory polymer. (b) Basic working mechanisms for the heating-responsive shape memory polymers. Reproduced with permission from [14], copyright reserved MDPI 2017.

2.2.1 SMPs Where the Switching Segment Is Based on Melting Temperature (T_m)

One way to fix the second phase of SMPs involves its crystallization, with the subsequent melting of this phase triggering shape recovery in the SMP. Typically, this category of materials includes chemically crosslinked semi-crystalline networks or (multi)block copolymers. Such materials exhibit higher stiffness than other SMPs and feature rapid shape recovery [13].

A significant portion of thermomechanical (TM)-type SMPs is composed of materials like polyolefins, polyethers, or polyesters, especially poly(ε-caprolactone). These "soft phases" possess low melting temperatures, allowing for the presence of a crystalline "hard phase" at the elevated switching temperature, a crucial feature for multi-block structures. Recently, a lot of researchers have paid significant attention to developing polyolefin-based elastomers. Zhang and coworkers showed the fabrication and metamorphism of biobased Eucommia ulmoides gum/polyolefin elastomer thermoplastic vulcanizates into a shape memory material exhibiting shape fixity and shape recovery above 95% [16]. Similarly, Zhu and coworkers developed multiple and reversible shape memory performances of polyolefin thermoplastic elastomer blends [17]. Figure 2.3 provides a visual representation of the one-way SME of the developed polyolefin thermoplastic elastomer blends. In this illustration, flat films labeled as E_1 and E_2 (while E_1 is a blend of Engage 8003/Infuse 9007/Engage 8180 = 30/40/30(%), E_2 is a blend of Engage 8003/Engage 8137/Engage 8180 = 30/30/40(%)) were created, with the edges of the E_1 sample marked in red and those of E_2 in green for ease of observation. As depicted in Figure 2.3a, an E_1 sample initially possessed a permanent flat shape and was heated to 85°C, where it was programmed into a temporary Shape 1 (resembling a "C" shape). Upon cooling to 50°C, Shape 1 was effectively fixed after removing the external force. In the subsequent step, E_1, now in Shape 1, was further programmed into a temporary Shape 2 (resembling a helix) at 50°C and then cooled to 0°C, firmly fixing the new temporary Shape 2. When E_1, now in Shape 2 at 0°C, was reheated to 50°C and then to 85°C, it rapidly transitioned back first to Shape 1 and then to the original permanent flat shape. Each of these shape transitions occurred within seconds.

Likewise, an E_2 sample demonstrated a similar capability to fix a temporary Shape 3 at 50°C and an additional temporary Shape 4 at 0°C. Upon heating, the sample in Shape 4 recovered to Shape 3 at 50°C and eventually returned to the permanent flat shape at 75°C. This series of transformations vividly showcases the one-way multi-SMEs exhibited by E_1 and E_2.

Another popular strategy to develop SMPs with crystalline switching temperature is by crosslinking low-density polyethylene (LDPE) with

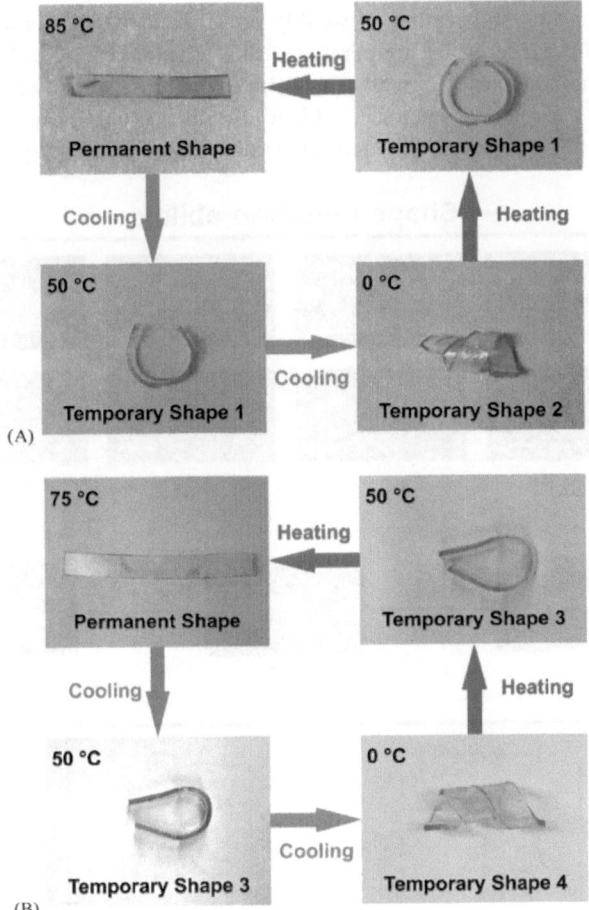

FIGURE 2.3   Multi-shape memory effects of (a) E_1 (polyolefin thermoplastic elastomer blends) at 0, 50, and 85°C and (b) E_2 at 0, 50, and 75°C. Reproduced with permission from [17], copyright reserved American Chemical Society 2019.

peroxides resulting in polymers that exhibit heat-induced shrinkage. The temperature required for this shrinkage can be adjusted by the stretch temperature applied, with higher stretch temperatures leading to higher shrinkage temperatures. The switching temperature can be widely tuned (ranging from 60°C to 100°C), depending on the degree of branching and crosslinking density, making this fabricating route a versatile way to develop semicrystalline SMPs [18]. Furthermore, natural rubber has been frequently used in SMP design, employing two distinct concepts. The first concept relies on strain-induced crystallization in weakly crosslinked (0.2%) natural rubber, which can be triggered by temperature, transversal stress, or solvent vapors [19]. The second approach involves crosslinked natural rubber with additives, such as fatty acids. For instance, a blend of natural rubber and stearic acid exhibits an SME based on the melting/crystallization of the fatty acid [20].

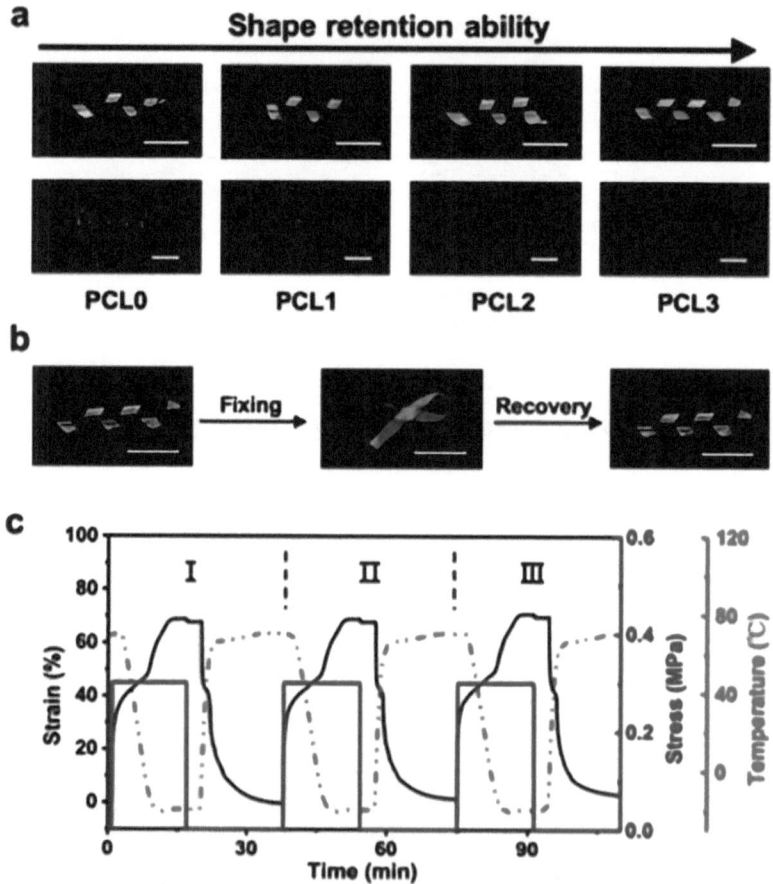

FIGURE 2.4 Demonstration of the shape-shifting behaviors. (a) Permanently reconfigured shapes for different samples. (b) Demonstration of the shape memory behavior for PCL (with butyl vinyl ether = 2 mol and polycaprolactone diacrylate 1.4 mol). (c) Consecutive shape memory cycles for PCL (with butyl vinyl ether = 2 mol and polycaprolactone diacrylate 1.4 mol). (All the scale bars are 10 mm). Reproduced with permission from [21], copyright reserved Royal Society of Chemistry 2020.

Low-melting aliphatic polyesters, particularly poly(ε-caprolactone) (PCL), are widely utilized as the "soft blocks" in SMPs (Figure 2.4) [21–23]. These soft blocks have found applications in various contexts, including polyurethane systems [24]. Furthermore, within the realm of SMPs, PCL-based formulations have been strategically enhanced by incorporating complementary materials like polyamides and polyaramides, which assume the role of "hard blocks" within these composite systems. This deliberate combination of PCL with such "hard blocks" introduces a synergistic approach to tailor the properties of SMPs. A pivotal characteristic that underscores the significance of PCL-based SMPs lies in their inherent tunability, particularly in terms of their switching temperature. This adaptability arises from the capacity to manipulate the molar mass of the polyester component. By precisely adjusting this parameter, it becomes entirely feasible to fine-tune the switching temperatures of these SMPs. This level of control extends to the ability to attain switching temperatures that closely align with physiological conditions, most notably the human body temperature, which typically hovers around 40°C (Figure 2.4). This precise control over switching temperatures enhances the applicability of PCL-based SMPs in contexts where responsiveness to physiological cues is paramount. In certain instances, crosslinked PCL has been harnessed as a highly effective and versatile SMP. This crosslinked form of PCL further extends the range of potential applications, showcasing the adaptability and utility of these materials in a variety of contexts and industries (Figure 2.4) [24].

2.2.2 SMPs Where the Switching Segment Is Based on Glass Transition Temperature (T_g)

SMPs with a switching segment based on melting temperature typically have a glass transition temperature below room temperature. Consequently, in the design of SMPs reliant on T_g activation, it is imperative to achieve an optimal T_g situated above room temperature. This ensures that these intelligent polymers can undergo shape programming without necessitating cryogenic cooling [25]. Diverging from SMPs predicated upon the melting temperature (T_M), those founded upon the glass transition temperature (Tg) manifest a discerning attribute: a comparatively protracted shape recovery process. This phenomenon can be ascribed to the inherent characteristic of the glass transition, which constitutes a second-order phase transition [26]. Consequently,

T_g-based SMPs may not be the optimal selection for applications necessitating expeditious and instantaneous shape restoration [26].

However, this characteristic, while seemingly a limitation in some scenarios, introduces an intriguing aspect that renders T_g-based SMPs particularly appealing in specific domains, most notably biomedical applications. The relatively slower shape recovery can be advantageous in such contexts, where controlled and gradual transformations are often preferred over sudden and abrupt changes. This attribute allows for a more controlled and precise response to stimuli, making T_g-based SMPs suitable candidates for a range of biomedical applications, where intricacy and precision are paramount considerations [1].

In the realm of SMPs, (meth)acrylate-based covalently crosslinked networks have risen to prominence (Figure 2.5). These networks primarily hinge upon the glass transition temperature (T_g) of the soft phase as the triggering mechanism for their shape memory attributes. Beyond their intriguing shape memory characteristics, these materials have garnered substantial attention for their potential utility in diverse bio applications. Among the notable qualities exhibited by these networks, some have demonstrated exceptional biocompatibility, rendering them well-suited for deployment in biomedical applications [27–29]. Concurrently, others have showcased inherent biodegradability, thus aligning with environmentally conscious considerations. Moreover, the structural framework of these methacrylate networks has been effectively translated into the creation of shape memory hydrogels, thereby expanding the realm of potential applications to encompass areas such as drug delivery systems, tissue engineering, and beyond [27–32].

The majority of SMPs, often categorized as "T_g-type" SMPs, typically possess transition temperatures well below 100°C [1]. However, a noteworthy exception exists in the domain of high-temperature SMPs, albeit such instances remain relatively scarce. For example, specific polyimides characterized by low crosslink densities have demonstrated remarkable switching temperatures, approximately 220°C (Figure 2.6). These polyimides exhibit notably swift recovery times, frequently on the order of seconds, coupled with shape fixity and recovery ratios surpassing 99%. Notably, these high-temperature SMPs offer a distinctive amalgamation of properties, including an exceptional room temperature storage modulus reaching values of up to 2,000 GPa, along with remarkable resistance to creep deformation [30].

These instances of high-temperature SMPs underscore the evolving landscape within the realm of SMPs. While the initial highlight of this field was primarily on applications characterized by lower switching temperatures,

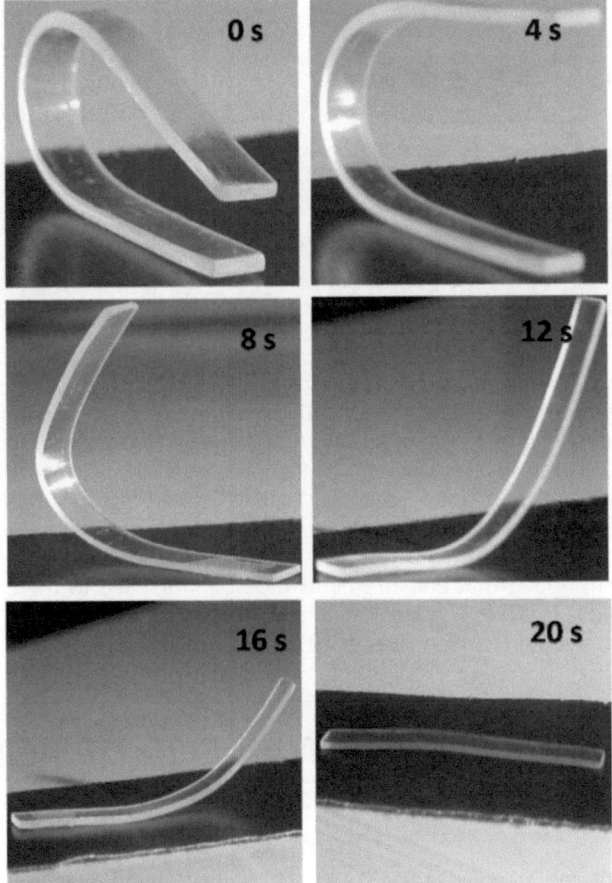

FIGURE 2.5 Thermoresponsive shape memory properties of poly(ethylene) glycol dimethacrylate-based shape memory polymer. Reproduced with permission from [30], copyright reserved Elsevier 2017.

particularly within the biomedical domain, it has progressively expanded its horizons into other sectors, encompassing domains such as aerospace applications [33]. This diversification underscores the growing versatility and potential of SMPs across various industries, wherein precise control over shape memory properties serves as a catalyst for innovation and technological advancements.

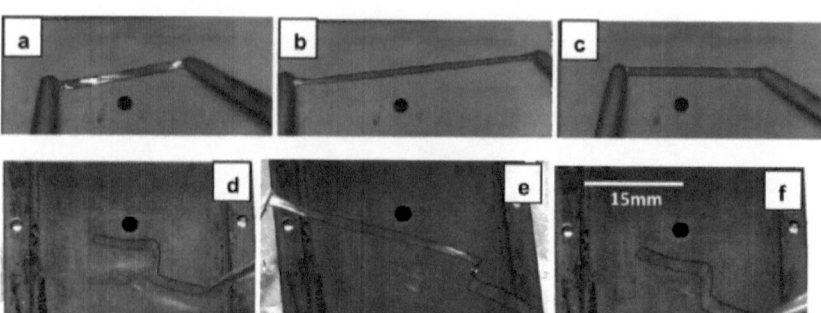

FIGURE 2.6 Shape recovery procedure of aromatic CP2 polyimide reinforced with single-wall carbon nanotube (SWNT) nanocomposites involving the use of a hotplate set to a temperature of 250 °C (shape recovery temperature). A sequence of images illustrates various phases of this process, beginning with the original state of the sample (a), followed by its stretched condition (b), subsequent relaxation (c), the introduction of a crease (d), elongation of the crease alongside it (e), and finally, the presence of a relaxed segment alongside an unaffected crease (f). It's worth noting that enhancements have been applied to the edges of the sample images to aid in visual clarity and guidance. Reproduced with permission from [31], copyright reserved Elsevier 2013.

2.3 GENERAL PATHWAY FOR DESIGNING LIGHT-RESPONSIVE (ONE-WAY) SMPS

Although thermoresponsive SMPs hold the highest share in terms of research and developmental output, the integration of light-responsive elements or molecules as molecular switches within polymer networks represents a significant breakthrough in the realm of material science [34]. This pioneering approach has laid the foundation for the creation of light-actuated shape memory or shape-changing polymer systems, ushering in a new era of innovative materials with remarkable capabilities. At the heart of this innovation lies the deliberate incorporation of light-sensitive moieties into precisely engineered polymer structures. This process is often complemented by a functionalization step, which fine-tunes the material's properties [35]. Together, these strategies bridge the gap between the molecular level, where light-induced effects originate, and the macroscopic scale, where these effects manifest themselves in visually perceptible ways. The outcome is a class of materials that can be dynamically and reversibly controlled by exposure to light, giving rise to a host of captivating light-induced properties [36].

In the realm of advanced materials, photosensitive shape memory polymers (PSMPs) exhibit a rich diversity, characterized by their unique capabilities and applications [34]. The classification of PSMPs into distinct categories is a notable facet of their versatility, with different criteria guiding their categorization. A particularly pertinent criterion is the wavelength of the actuating light, which has led to the division of PSMPs into three primary categories: ultraviolet light (UV), visible light (VIS), and infrared light (IR). Each of these categories possesses distinctive attributes and functionalities, as outlined below.

PSMPs responsive to UV light are renowned for their exceptional photoresponsive properties. These materials undergo structural alterations when exposed to UV radiation, enabling changes in shape or properties (Figure 2.7). This category holds significant value in applications necessitating precise and expeditious actuation, given that UV light serves as a potent energy source for initiating these materials. UV-responsive PSMPs find valuable roles in domains such as microelectronics, optics, and photonics, where rapid and intricate changes in shape or properties are paramount. Similarly, PSMPs activated by VIS light occupy a prominent position, primarily owing to the ubiquity of VIS light sources. This category encompasses a broad spectrum of wavelengths within the VIS range, rendering it adaptable

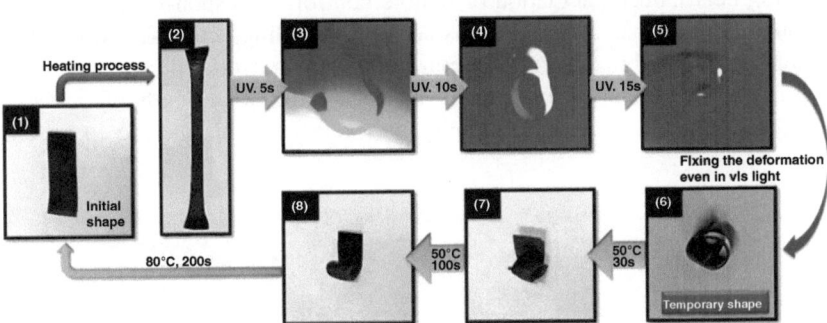

FIGURE 2.7 Staging-responsive SMPs. Shape memory polymers based on N-Methyldiethanolamine (MDEA) and 4,4-azodibenzoic acid polyurethanes were heated to 100°C and stretched to 100% strain with a rate of 20 mm min^{-1}. The sample was subsequently cooled to room temperature to achieve the treated shape (2). The treated sample curled quickly under UV irradiation (3–5). The deformed shape was fixed after ending UV irradiation, and the temporary shape was unchanged even in VIS light (5–6). Upon heating, the temporary shape was recovered sequentially at 50°C (6–8). The initial shape (1) was recovered at 80°C. Reproduced with permission from [37], copyright reserved Royal Society of Chemistry 2017.

to diverse illumination conditions. VIS-responsive PSMPs find relevance in scenarios demanding controlled and reversible shape alterations or mechanical responses. For instance, in the realm of smart materials and consumer electronics, these materials prove invaluable for optical devices and sensors, capable of responding to ambient lighting conditions [37].

Furthermore, PSMPs designed to react to IR light stand out for their ability to respond to longer wavelengths, often associated with heat. These materials exhibit shape changes or property adjustments upon exposure to IR radiation. For example, Lan and his research team undertook the development of a styrene-based SMP, a significant endeavor in the realm of materials science. Their pioneering work not only resulted in the creation of this innovative polymer but also served as a demonstrative platform for the activation of SMPs through the utilization of medium-IR laser light (Figure 2.8) [38]. The methodology employed by Lan et al. involved the transmission of medium-IR light via an optical fiber that was intricately embedded within the SMP matrix. This approach enabled precise and controlled activation of the SMP using laser light within the medium-IR spectrum. Notably, the implementation of medium-IR light as the triggering mechanism showcases the team's forward-thinking approach, capitalizing on the unique properties of this specific light range (Figure 2.8) [38].

This category assumes particular significance in applications necessitating heat-induced actuation or remote control. IR-responsive PSMPs have found applications across various sectors, including aerospace, where they are instrumental in adaptive structures and mechanisms.

The classification of PSMPs based on the wavelength of actuating light underscores their adaptability and versatility in catering to specific

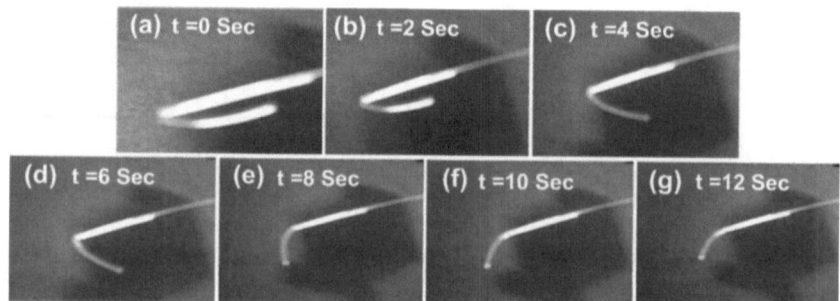

FIGURE 2.8 Shape recovery snapshots of the SMP induced by infrared light. (a) Initial predeformed configuration. (b)–(g) Deployment sequence of the actuator at t = 2, 4, 6, 8, 10, and 12 s, respectively. Reproduced with permission from [38], copyright reserved AIP 2010.

application requirements. These smart polymers are engineered to harness the unique attributes of different segments of the electromagnetic spectrum, thereby providing tailored solutions across a diverse array of industries and technologies. The capability to precisely govern shape changes, mechanical responses, or property modifications in response to varied light sources holds immense promise, propelling advancements in fields ranging from materials science to engineering and beyond. This paradigm shift has opened up an exciting avenue for the development of materials that respond to external stimuli with unparalleled precision. These materials can change shape, structure, or properties upon exposure to light, offering a wide range of potential applications across various industries, from optoelectronics to biomedical devices. The ability to harness light as a trigger for macroscopic changes has unlocked new possibilities in material science, promising to redefine the way we design and utilize advanced materials in the future [39,40].

One notable advantage of light-responsive polymers, particularly in contrast to their thermally driven shape memory polymer counterparts, is the ability to initiate the SME independently of temperature variations [41]. This intrinsic feature allows for precise and controlled activation through exposure to light. Furthermore, the reversibility of light-induced shape changes is a defining characteristic of these polymers. Upon removal of the light source, these materials seamlessly revert to their original shape, demonstrating their versatility and potential for various applications [42].

The light response in these polymers can manifest in two primary forms: photochemical and photothermal. The photochemical effect hinges on photoreactions of light-sensitive groups, such as photoisomerization and photodimerization, wherein chemical reactions power and govern mechanical motion (Figure 2.9). Conversely, the photothermal effect involves the conversion of light into heat, which, in turn, drives mechanical work. Both of these fundamental concepts have found practical application in the realm of light-responsive polymer systems [34].

The procedure for photothermal staged-responsive shape memory of the prepared polyurethane is outlined in Figure 2.9g [34]. Finally, Figure 2.9h presents a sequence of events where Sample (1) is heated to 100°C, stretched to 100% strain, and cooled to room temperature and subsequently curls quickly under UV irradiation. The deformed shape is fixed after UV irradiation, and the temporary shape remains unchanged even in VIS. Upon heating, the temporary shape sequentially recovers at 50°C, ultimately restoring the initial shape at 80°C [34].

In recent years, the landscape of materials science has witnessed a remarkable proliferation of light-driven polymeric materials, representing a diverse and dynamic array of innovations. This burgeoning field encompasses a wide spectrum of polymer classes, including liquid crystalline polymeric

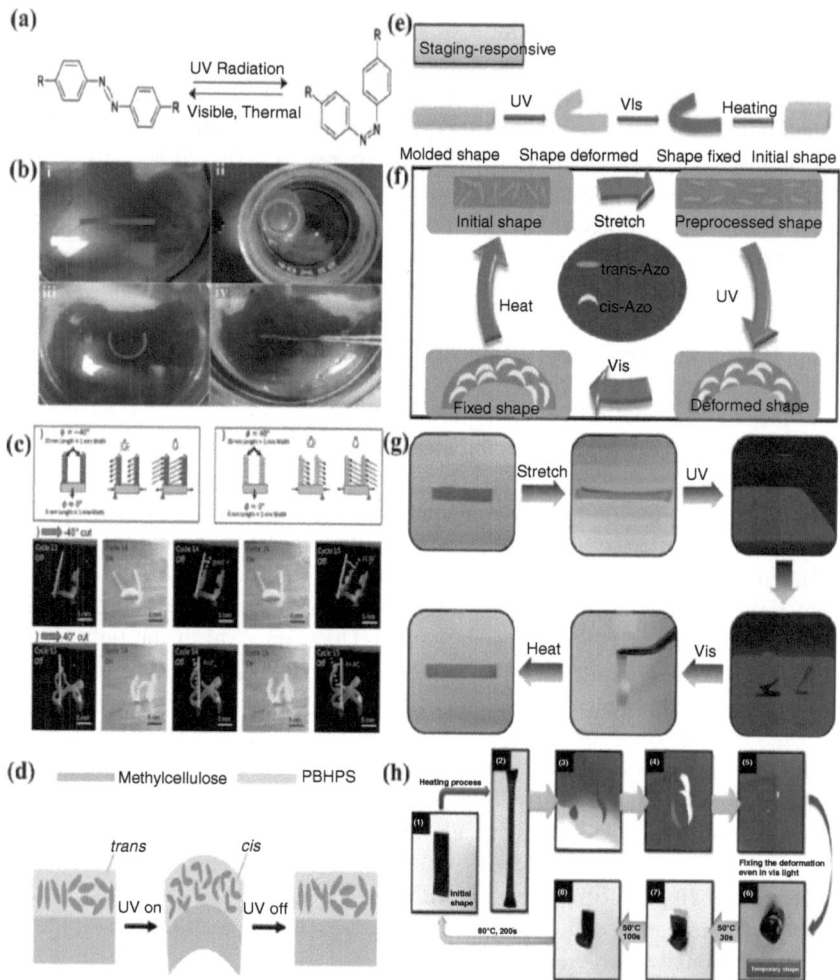

FIGURE 2.9 Depiction of a series of illustrations and schematics outlining various photoresponsive phenomena and shape memory effects. In (a), azobenzene-based molecules exhibit E-Z isomerization upon exposure to UV/VIS radiation. Moving to (b), the photoresponsive shape memory effect of αCD-Alg/Azo-PAA film is showcased, with stages showing the original shape, deformed shape, temporary shape, and recovered shape. In (c), two cycles are illustrated, accompanied by the clockwise rotation of the legs at an angle of −40° (or 40°). Figure (d) provides a schematic representation of the light-driven deformation of the P/MC film with the UV on or off. In (e), the working principle of the staging-responsive SMP is illustrated. (f) elucidates the mechanism behind the photothermal staged-responsive shape memory properties at the molecular level. Reproduced with permission from [34], copyright reserved Elsevier 2022.

(LCP) materials [43–46], hydrogels [47], and shape memory composites [35]. These polymers exhibit a broad range of characteristics, spanning from semi-crystalline to amorphous in nature, and they have been skillfully molded into various initial shapes, spanning from films and fibers to tubes. The driving force behind these extensive developments is the pursuit of materials that can seamlessly transition between different shapes and configurations under the influence of light. This transformative capability is a hallmark of these materials and holds tremendous potential for a multitude of applications.

LCP materials, for instance, exhibit complex and tunable optical properties, making them invaluable in fields such as optics and photonics. Hydrogels, with their high-water content and biocompatibility, are being explored for applications in drug delivery systems and tissue engineering, promising advancements in the biomedical domain. Shape memory polymers, whether semicrystalline or amorphous, are being employed in various sectors, including aerospace and automotive industries, to create adaptive and responsive components [48,49]. These materials have not only expanded the materials science toolkit but have also ushered in an era of reconfigurable systems with the ability to undergo shape changes on demand. By offering a versatile platform for materials engineering, these advancements are set to redefine the boundaries of what is achievable in fields ranging from optics to biomedicine [48,49].

2.4 GENERAL PATHWAY FOR DESIGNING MAGNETIC-RESPONSIVE (ONE-WAY) SMPS

In the ever-evolving landscape of materials science, magnetic shape memory polymers (MSMPs) and magnetic shape memory materials (MSMs) have emerged as compelling frontiers that break away from the conventional paradigms of shape memory materials [50]. These innovative materials not only introduce novel capabilities but also offer a distinctive perspective on how SMEs can be harnessed, setting them apart from their traditional temperature-responsive counterparts. Traditionally, when we think of shape memory materials, the immediate association is with temperature-induced transformations [51]. However, the advent of MSMs represents a paradigm shift, as they pivot toward an entirely new mode of activation, one that centers around the manipulation of magnetic fields as the driving force for shape transitions.

This departure from the conventional temperature-based activation is a hallmark of MSMPs and MSMs, marking a significant departure from the well-established norm. These materials embrace magnetic fields as the stimulus for shaping memory responses, a departure that brings forth a range of opportunities and applications in diverse domains. For example, Sang et al. demonstrated that incorporating magneto-responsive SMPs into 4D printing enables the creation of intelligent products with contactless control [52]. Their study developed robust SMPs with magneto-responsive properties using a blend of polylactic acid (PLA), thermoplastic polyurethane (TPU), and Fe_3O_4 particles for 3D printing. The resulting PLA/TPU/Fe_3O_4 material exhibited strong tensile properties, uniform magnetic particle distribution, and rapid magnetic response, making it highly efficient in heat generation. Smart structures, including a honeycomb and bionic flower-like model, were designed and printed. These structures, when subjected to external forces, could completely recover their original shape under a contactless magnetic field (Figure 2.10).

In essence, MSMPs and MSMs represent a forward-looking direction in materials science, one that challenges preconceived notions and explores the uncharted territories of magnetic-driven SMEs. This pioneering approach not only expands the scope of shape memory materials but also ushers in new possibilities for innovative solutions and applications in a wide array of industries, from biomedicine to materials engineering [53]. As we delve deeper into the intricacies of these materials, we unlock the potential to reshape the future of materials research and development, paving the way for dynamic, adaptable, and responsive materials with multifaceted applications. In the biomedical domain, there is a growing interest in MSMs, primarily because they eliminate the need for external heat sources, enhancing their safety and minimizing the invasiveness associated with introducing heat into the body [53]. Moreover, the capacity for internal heating holds promise for applications in various domains, such as expediting the curing process of thermoset adhesives, achieved through induction heating of magnetic particles under an alternating current (AC) field.

Generally speaking, MSMPs and MSMs both share a common foundation: a polymer or elastomer matrix embedded with magnetic particles that play a pivotal role in inducing SMEs when exposed to external magnetic fields [54]. Despite this commonality, the distinction between these two materials lies in how the embedded magnetic particles trigger the shape-changing process [54].

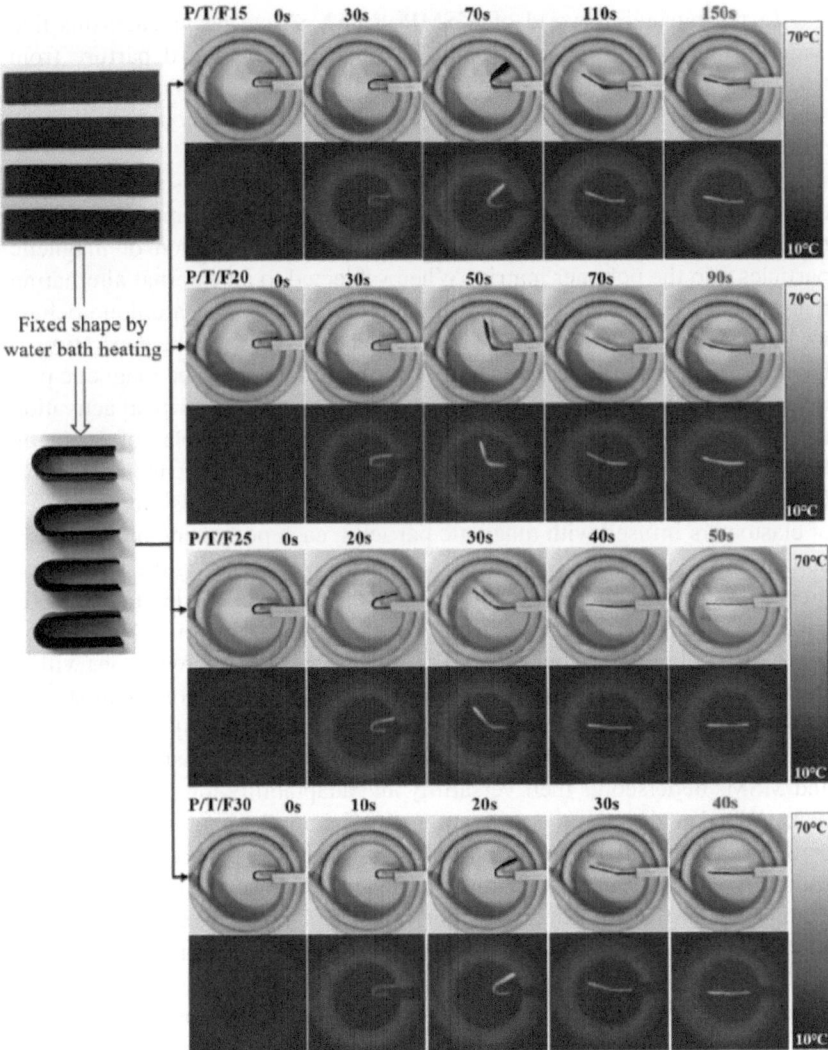

FIGURE 2.10   Shape memory behavior of the composites with different Fe_3O_4 contents triggered by the magnetic field. Reproduced with permission from [52], copyright reserved Elsevier 2023.

In the intriguing world of MSMPs and MSMs), the mechanisms that underlie their shape-changing abilities offer a fascinating departure from traditional shape memory materials. These materials introduce innovative approaches to trigger shape transitions, diverging from the conventional reliance on temperature changes [55].

Within the realm of MSMPs, these are essentially SMPs that have been enhanced with the capability to respond to heat as the primary triggering mechanism. The key feature lies in the strategic integration of magnetic particles into the polymer matrix. When subjected to an external alternating magnetic field, these embedded magnetic particles exhibit a unique behavior known as induction heating. This phenomenon involves the generation of localized temperature increases within the material due to the magnetic particles heating up. As the material's temperature reaches the critical activation threshold, the SME is set into motion. This intricate interplay of magnetic field-induced heating ultimately leads to the desired shape change [56–58]. In contrast, MSMs take a distinct approach. These materials are composed of elastomers infused with magnetic particles, each possessing precise magnetization patterns that are meticulously incorporated during the fabrication process. When introduced into an external static magnetic field, the magnetic particles within the material dutifully align themselves with the orientation of the external magnetic field. This alignment generates micro torques within the elastomer matrix, effectively creating forces that act upon the material, compelling it to conform to a pre-programmed shape [56–58].

This fundamental distinction in the activation mechanisms of MSMPs and MSMs underscores their versatility and adaptability for diverse applications. Whether through the utilization of induction heating within MSMPs or the alignment of magnetic particles within MSMs, these materials are endowed with the remarkable ability to undergo precise and reversible shape changes under the influence of magnetic fields. This innovative approach to shape memory materials opens a world of possibilities, offering solutions for a wide array of industries, from biomedicine to materials engineering, where controlled and non-invasive shape transitions are of paramount importance. The advent of MSMPs and MSMs paves the way for pioneering advancements that are poised to redefine the landscape of shape memory materials research and application.

The exploration of MSMPs and MSMs showcases their potential in a wide array of applications where controlled shape changes or deformations are prerequisites [59–61]. These materials not only offer the unique advantage of remote controllability but also provide a non-invasive means of activation, making them promising candidates in fields ranging from biomedicine to materials engineering. The capacity to harness magnetic fields for precise and reversible shape changes has the potential to revolutionize the landscape of shape memory materials research and application, introducing innovative solutions and opportunities in the ever-evolving domain of materials science and engineering [59–61].

2.5 GENERAL PATHWAY FOR DESIGNING SOLVENT-RESPONSIVE (ONE-WAY) SMPS

Figure 2.11 serves as an illuminating visual aid that provides a comprehensive understanding of how solvents play a pivotal role in shaping the shape memory mechanisms inherent to both amorphous and semicrystalline SMPs. Traditionally, SMPs have been primarily activated by thermal stimuli, necessitating the material to be heated beyond its specific transition temperature, such as T_g (glass transition temperature) for amorphous polymers or T_m (melting temperature) for semicrystalline ones. This thermal activation prompts the network to gracefully revert to its original, undeformed state, embodying the core principle of shape memory materials.

However, the introduction of solvents into the realm of SMPs ushers in a fascinating and distinctive dimension. Instead of undergoing a complete return to the original shape, the material exhibits a remarkable behavior – it reverts to an intermediate shape, diverging from the permanent form. This intermediate shape possesses a pliable and malleable quality, and the transition between this intermediate state and the permanent shape is orchestrated by a dynamic interplay of swelling and deswelling processes, intricately guided by the interactions between the polymer matrix and the solvent molecules. Notably, the choice of solvent used in this process assumes a critical role as it directly influences the extent of swelling and deswelling within the material, thereby wielding significant control over the ensuing recovery process.

In essence, Figure 2.11 encapsulates the essence of how solvents introduce a transformative facet to SMPs, making them responsive to a unique set of stimuli. This visual representation underscores the dynamic and versatile nature of shape memory materials, showcasing their adaptability to diverse environmental conditions and their potential for a wide array of applications, ranging from biomedical devices to responsive structures [62].

In our prior correspondence [63], we engaged in a detailed exploration of various constitutive models that elucidate the impact of solvents on the thermomechanical characteristics of amorphous networks (Tg-based systems), ultimately bolstering the shape recovery process. As a broad consensus, solvents have been consistently demonstrated to augment chain mobility, consequently heightening the overall configurational entropy within the system.

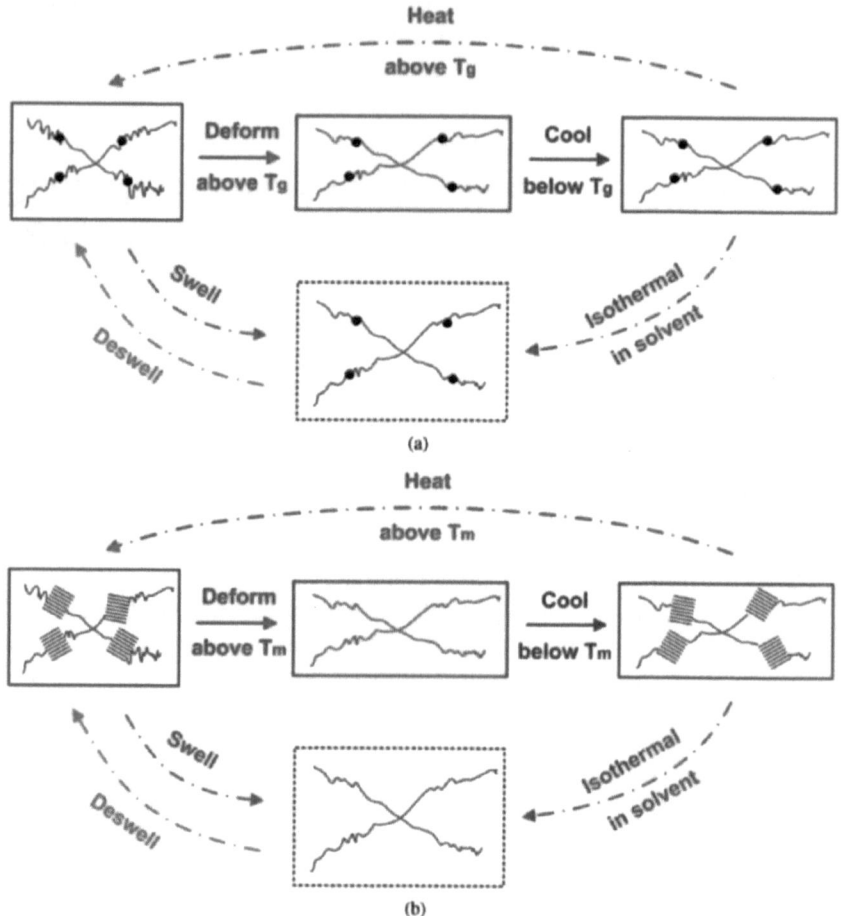

FIGURE 2.11 The physical mechanism behind heating and solvent-responsive SMPs: (a) amorphous polymers and (b) semicrystalline polymers. Reproduced with permission from [62], copyright reserved Wiley 2020.

This, in turn, leads to a reduction in the relaxation time and a lowering of the glass transition temperature, a phenomenon that finds resonance with the renowned Adam-Gibbs model [63].

Similarly, in the realm of semicrystalline-based SMPs, solvent-induced recovery introduces a fascinating and distinct mechanism compared to its amorphous counterparts. The crucial role of the solvent in this context lies in its ability to dissolve the crystalline segments within the polymer matrix. This dissolution initiates a cascade of events that lead to the recovery of the polymer's original shape, as visually represented in Figure 2.11.

A notable study by Loh and collaborators exemplifies the innovative approach to designing solvent-responsive SMPs. Their work involves a carefully engineered blend of poly(ethylene glycol) (PEG), poly(ε-caprolactone) (PCL), and poly(dimethylsiloxane) (PDMS). Within this unique composite material, the solvation of PEG domains plays a pivotal role in achieving shape recovery [64].

An intriguing revelation stemming from the thermal analysis conducted in this study sheds light on the relationship between the presence of PEG (polyethylene glycol) segments and the crystallinity of the polymer matrix. It's observed that the incorporation of a relatively small amount of PEG (7 wt%) results in modest crystallinity, measured at 0.8%. Conversely, a higher content of PEG (28.9 wt%) significantly elevates the crystallinity to 6.6% [64]. This increase in PEG domains brings about several notable advantages to the SMP system (Figure 2.12).

Firstly, the heightened presence of PEG enhances the fixity of the material, implying that the temporary shape is better retained during deformation. Secondly, it facilitates the recovery process, enabling the material to return to its permanent shape more efficiently. These enhancements are attributed to the reinforced fixing network within the polymer matrix due to the increased presence of PEG domains, consequently amplifying the stored energy available for the recovery process [62].

The correlation between PEG content and crystallinity underscores the pivotal role of PEG in dictating the mechanical properties and shape memory behavior of the polymer. Understanding and leveraging this relationship could

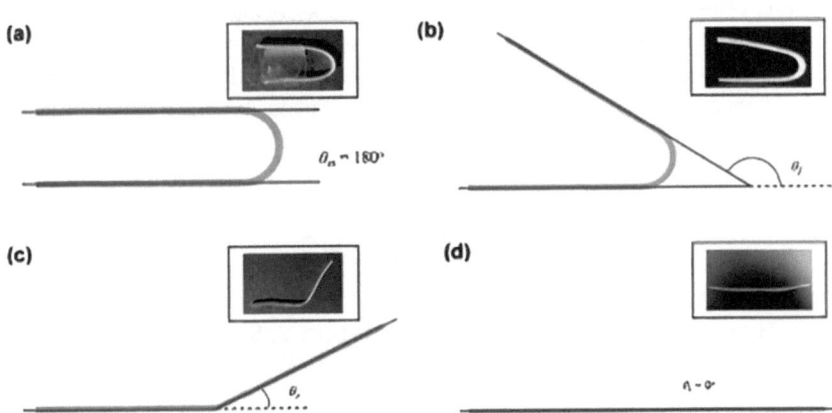

FIGURE 2.12 Schematic illustration of the characterization of the shape memory effect (SME) triggered by water. (a) Determination of the maximum deformation angle, (b) assessment of the fixity angle, and (c) and (d) measurement of the recovery angle. Reproduced with permission from [64], copyright reserved Royal Society of Chemistry 2017.

potentially lead to the development of tailored SMP systems with enhanced performance and functionality for various applications.

In the realm of semicrystalline polymers, it's imperative to recognize the intimate relationship between the efficiency and duration of the shape recovery process and the diffusion coefficient of the solvent [63,64]. Put simply, the speed at which the crystalline domains of these polymers are solvated directly influences how swiftly they regain their original shape. This underscores the critical importance of comprehending the intricate interplay between solvent properties and the behavior of SMPs within semicrystalline systems.

A key insight derived from this relationship is that a faster solvation process of the crystalline domains corresponds to a more rapid shape recovery. This knowledge opens up intriguing possibilities for manipulating these interactions to engineer smart materials with precise control over their shape memory capabilities in response to solvent stimuli [65,66]. By fine-tuning the properties of the solvent and understanding its influence on the polymer matrix, researchers can effectively modulate the shape memory behavior of SMPs in semicrystalline systems.

This capability holds tremendous promise for the development of advanced materials with tailored responses to specific environmental cues. For instance, by designing SMPs that exhibit rapid shape recovery in response to particular solvents, researchers can create smart materials suited for applications where quick and precise shape changes are desired. Such materials could find utility in diverse fields, including responsive textiles, biomedical devices, and adaptive structures. Furthermore, the ability to customize the solvent-polymer interactions offers a pathway to address challenges associated with conventional shape memory materials. By overcoming limitations related to shape recovery timescales and efficiency, tailored solvent-responsive SMPs could pave the way for enhanced performance and functionality in various practical applications.

REFERENCES

1. Hager, M. D., Bode, S., Weber, C., & Schubert, U. S. (2015). Shape memory polymers: Past, present and future developments. *Progress in Polymer Science, 49*, 3–33.
2. Leonardi, A. B., Fasce, L. A., Zucchi, I. A., Hoppe, C. E., Soulé, E. R., Pérez, C. J., & Williams, R. J. (2011). Shape memory epoxies based on networks with chemical and physical crosslinks. *European Polymer Journal, 47*(3), 362–369.
3. Barot, G., Rao, I. J., & Rajagopal, K. R. (2008). A thermodynamic framework for the modeling of crystallizable shape memory polymers. *International Journal of Engineering Science, 46*(4), 325–351.

4. Liu, G., Ding, X., Cao, Y., Zheng, Z., & Peng, Y. (2005). Novel shape-memory polymer with two transition temperatures. *Macromolecular Rapid Communications, 26*(8), 649–652.

5. Basak, S., Dasgupta, P., & Bandyopadhyay, A. (2023). One-way shape memory polyesters-evolution, growth, developments, and current trends. *Polymer-Plastics Technology and Materials, 62*(17), 2286–2317.

6. Guo, B., Chen, Y., Lei, Y., Zhang, L., Zhou, W. Y., Rabie, A. B. M., & Zhao, J. (2011). Biobased poly (propylene sebacate) as shape memory polymer with tunable switching temperature for potential biomedical applications. *Biomacromolecules, 12*(4), 1312–1321.

7. Bao, M., Lou, X., Zhou, Q., Dong, W., Yuan, H., & Zhang, Y. (2014). Electrospun biomimetic fibrous scaffold from shape memory polymer of PDLLA-co-TMC for bone tissue engineering. *ACS Applied Materials & Interfaces, 6*(4), 2611–2621.

8. Yang, J., Zhao, W., Yang, Z., He, W., Wang, J., Ikeda, T., & Jiang, L. (2019). Photonic shape memory polymer based on liquid crystalline blue phase films. *ACS Applied Materials & Interfaces, 11*(49), 46124–46131.

9. Benkhaled, B. T., Belkhir, K., Brossier, T., Chatard, C., Graillot, A., Lonetti, B., ... & Lapinte, V. (2022). 3D fabrication of shape-memory polymer networks based on coumarin photo-dimerization. *European Polymer Journal, 179*, 111570.

10. Zhang, G., Zhao, Q., Yang, L., Zou, W., Xi, X., & Xie, T. (2016). Exploring dynamic equilibrium of Diels–Alder reaction for solid state plasticity in remoldable shape memory polymer network. *ACS Macro Letters, 5*(7), 805–808.

11. Lu, W., Le, X., Zhang, J., Huang, Y., & Chen, T. (2017). Supramolecular shape memory hydrogels: A new bridge between stimuli-responsive polymers and supramolecular chemistry. *Chemical Society Reviews, 46*(5), 1284–1294.

12. Leng, J., Lan, X., Liu, Y., & Du, S. (2011). Shape-memory polymers and their composites: Stimulus methods and applications. *Progress in Materials Science, 56*(7), 1077–1135.

13. Liu, C., Qin, H., & Mather, P. T. (2007). Review of progress in shape-memory polymers. *Journal of Materials Chemistry, 17*(16), 1543–1558.

14. Wu, X., Huang, W. M., Zhao, Y., Ding, Z., Tang, C., & Zhang, J. (2013). Mechanisms of the shape memory effect in polymeric materials. *Polymers, 5*(4), 1169–1202.

15. Basak, S., & Bandyopadhyay, A. (2022). Two-way semicrystalline shape memory elastomers: Development and current research trends. *Advanced Engineering Materials, 24*(10), 2200257.

16. Kang, H., Gong, M., Xu, M., Wang, H., Li, Y., Fang, Q., & Zhang, L. (2019). Fabricated biobased Eucommia ulmoides gum/polyolefin elastomer thermoplastic vulcanizates into a shape memory material. *Industrial & Engineering Chemistry Research, 58*(16), 6375–6384.

17. Gao, Y., Liu, W., & Zhu, S. (2019). Thermoplastic polyolefin elastomer blends for multiple and reversible shape memory polymers. *Industrial & Engineering Chemistry Research, 58*(42), 19495–19502.

18. Zhao, J., Chen, M., Wang, X., Zhao, X., Wang, Z., Dang, Z. M., ... & Chen, F. (2013). Triple shape memory effects of cross-linked polyethylene/polypropylene blends with cocontinuous architecture. *ACS Applied Materials & Interfaces, 5*(12), 5550–5556.

19. Quitmann, D., Reinders, F. M., Heuwers, B., Katzenberg, F., & Tiller, J. C. (2015). Programming of shape memory natural rubber for near-discrete shape transitions. *ACS Applied Materials & Interfaces*, *7*(3), 1486–1490.

20. Du, J., Liu, D., Zhang, Z., Yao, X., Wan, D., Pu, H., & Lu, Z. (2017). Dual-responsive triple-shape memory polyolefin elastomer/stearic acid composite. *Polymer*, *126*, 206–210.

21. Miao, W., Zou, W., Luo, Y., Zheng, N., Zhao, Q., & Xie, T. (2020). Structural tuning of polycaprolactone based thermadapt shape memory polymer. *Polymer Chemistry*, *11*(7), 1369–1374.

22. Bai, Y., Jiang, C., Wang, Q., & Wang, T. (2013). A novel high mechanical strength shape memory polymer based on ethyl cellulose and polycaprolactone. *Carbohydrate Polymers*, *96*(2), 522–527.

23. Joo, Y. S., Cha, J. R., & Gong, M. S. (2018). Biodegradable shape-memory polymers using polycaprolactone and isosorbide based polyurethane blends. *Materials Science and Engineering: C*, *91*, 426–435.

24. Huang, W. M., Yang, B., & Fu, Y. Q. (2011). *Polyurethane shape memory polymers*. CRC Press.

25. Hockings, N., Iravani, P., & Bowen, C. R. (2014, November). Artificial ligamentous joints: Methods, materials and characteristics. In *2014 IEEE-RAS International Conference on Humanoid Robots* (pp. 20–26). IEEE.

26. Ahmad, M., Luo, J., Xu, B., Purnawali, H., King, P. J., Chalker, P. R., ... & Miraftab, M. (2011). Synthesis and characterization of polyurethane-based shape-memory polymers for tailored Tg around body temperature for medical applications. *Macromolecular Chemistry and Physics*, *212*(6), 592–602.

27. Hu, J., Zhu, Y., Huang, H., & Lu, J. (2012). Recent advances in shape–memory polymers: Structure, mechanism, functionality, modeling and applications. *Progress in Polymer Science*, *37*(12), 1720–1763.

28. Ge, Q., Sakhaei, A. H., Lee, H., Dunn, C. K., Fang, N. X., & Dunn, M. L. (2016). Multimaterial 4D printing with tailorable shape memory polymers. *Scientific Reports*, *6*(1), 31110.

29. Capiel, G., Marcovich, N. E., & Mosiewicki, M. A. (2019). Shape memory polymer networks based on methacrylated fatty acids. *European Polymer Journal*, *116*, 321–329.

30. Antony, G. J. M., Jarali, C. S., Aruna, S. T., & Raja, S. (2017). Tailored poly (ethylene) glycol dimethacrylate based shape memory polymer for orthopedic applications. *Journal of the Mechanical Behavior of Biomedical Materials*, *65*, 857–865.

31. Koerner, H., Strong, R. J., Smith, M. L., Wang, D. H., Tan, L. S., Lee, K. M., ... & Vaia, R. A. (2013). Polymer design for high temperature shape memory: Low crosslink density polyimides. *Polymer*, *54*(1), 391–402.

32. Yoonessi, M., Shi, Y., Scheiman, D. A., Lebron-Colon, M., Tigelaar, D. M., Weiss, R. A., & Meador, M. A. (2012). Graphene polyimide nanocomposites; thermal, mechanical, and high-temperature shape memory effects. *ACS Nano*, *6*(9), 7644–7655.

33. Li, F., Liu, Y., & Leng, J. (2019). Progress of shape memory polymers and their composites in aerospace applications. *Smart Materials and Structures*, *28*(10), 103003.

34. Wang, Y., Wang, Y., Wei, Q., & Zhang, J. (2022). Light-responsive shape memory polymer composites. *European Polymer Journal, 173,* 111314.
35. Meng, H., & Li, G. (2013). A review of stimuli-responsive shape memory polymer composites. *Polymer, 54*(9), 2199–2221.
36. Chen, Y., Zhao, X., Luo, C., Shao, Y., Yang, M. B., & Yin, B. (2020). A facile fabrication of shape memory polymer nanocomposites with fast light-response and self-healing performance. *Composites Part A: Applied Science and Manufacturing, 135,* 105931.
37. Ban, J., Mu, L., Yang, J., Chen, S., & Zhuo, H. (2017). New stimulus-responsive shape-memory polyurethanes capable of UV light-triggered deformation, hydrogen bond-mediated fixation, and thermal-induced recovery. *Journal of Materials Chemistry A, 5*(28), 14514–14518.
38. Leng, J., Zhang, D., Liu, Y., Yu, K., & Lan, X. (2010). Study on the activation of styrene-based shape memory polymer by medium-infrared laser light. *Applied Physics Letters, 96*(11), 111905.
39. Xu, J., & Song, J. (2011). Thermal responsive shape memory polymers for biomedical applications. *Biomedical Engineering-Frontiers and Challenges,* 125–142.
40. Fang, L., Fang, T., Liu, X., Ni, Y., Lu, C., & Xu, Z. (2017). Precise stimulation of near-infrared light responsive shape-memory polymer composites using upconversion particles with photothermal capability. *Composites Science and Technology, 152,* 190–197.
41. Stoychev, G., Kirillova, A., & Ionov, L. (2019). Light-responsive shape-changing polymers. *Advanced Optical Materials, 7*(16), 1900067.
42. Zhu, Y., & Egap, E. (2021). Light-mediated polymerization induced by semiconducting nanomaterials: State-of-the-art and future perspectives. *ACS Polymers Au, 1*(2), 76–99.
43. Mehta, K., Peeketi, A. R., Liu, L., Broer, D., Onck, P., & Annabattula, R. K. (2020). Design and applications of light responsive liquid crystal polymer thin films. *Appl. Phys. Rev. 7,* 041306 (2020); https://doi.org/10.1063/5.0014619.
44. Liu, Y., Wu, W., Wei, J., & Yu, Y. (2017). Visible light responsive liquid crystal polymers containing reactive moieties with good processability. *ACS Applied Materials & Interfaces, 9*(1), 782–789.
45. Da Cunha, M. P., Debije, M. G., & Schenning, A. P. (2020). Bioinspired light-driven soft robots based on liquid crystal polymers. *Chemical Society Reviews, 49*(18), 6568–6578.
46. Wei, J., & Yu, Y. (2012). Photodeformable polymer gels and crosslinked liquid-crystalline polymers. *Soft Matter, 8*(31), 8050–8059.
47. Jiang, Z., Tan, M. L., Taheri, M., Yan, Q., Tsuzuki, T., Gardiner, M. G., ... & Connal, L. A. (2020). Strong, self-healable, and recyclable visible-light-responsive hydrogel actuators. *Angewandte Chemie, 132*(18), 7115–7122.
48. Kirillova, A., & Ionov, L. (2019). Shape-changing polymers for biomedical applications. *Journal of Materials Chemistry B, 7*(10), 1597–1624.
49. Li, Q., Schenning, A. P., & Bunning, T. J. (2019). Light-responsive smart soft matter technologies. *Advanced Optical Materials, 7*(16), 1901160.
50. Hassan, R. U., Jo, S., & Seok, J. (2018). Fabrication of a functionally graded and magnetically responsive shape memory polymer using a 3 D printing technique and its characterization. *Journal of Applied Polymer Science, 135*(11), 45997.

51. Baniasadi, M., Yarali, E., Bodaghi, M., Zolfagharian, A., & Baghani, M. (2021). Constitutive modeling of multi-stimuli-responsive shape memory polymers with multi-functional capabilities. *International Journal of Mechanical Sciences*, *192*, 106082.

52. Liu, H., Wang, F., Wu, W., Dong, X., & Sang, L. (2023). 4D printing of mechanically robust PLA/TPU/Fe3O4 magneto-responsive shape memory polymers for smart structures. *Composites Part B: Engineering*, *248*, 110382.

53. Leungpuangkaew, S., Amornkitbamrung, L., Phetnoi, N., Sapcharoenkun, C., Jubsilp, C., Ekgasit, S., & Rimdusit, S. (2023). Magnetic-and light-responsive shape memory polymer nanocomposites from bio-based benzoxazine resin and iron oxide nanoparticles. *Advanced Industrial and Engineering Polymer Research*, *6*(3), 215–225.

54. van Vilsteren, S. J., Yarmand, H., & Ghodrat, S. (2021). Review of magnetic shape memory polymers and magnetic soft materials. *Magnetochemistry*, *7*(9), 123.

55. Yue, C., Li, M., Liu, Y., Fang, Y., Song, Y., Xu, M., & Li, J. (2021). Three-dimensional printing of cellulose nanofibers reinforced PHB/PCL/Fe3O4 magneto-responsive shape memory polymer composites with excellent mechanical properties. *Additive Manufacturing*, *46*, 102146.

56. Meng, H., Mohamadian, H., Stubblefield, M., Jerro, D., Ibekwe, S., Pang, S. S., & Li, G. (2013). Various shape memory effects of stimuli-responsive shape memory polymers. *Smart Materials and Structures*, *22*(9), 093001.

57. Du, L., Xu, Z. Y., Fan, C. J., Xiang, G., Yang, K. K., & Wang, Y. Z. (2018). A fascinating metallo-supramolecular polymer network with thermal/magnetic/light-responsive shape-memory effects anchored by Fe3O4 nanoparticles. *Macromolecules*, *51*(3), 705–715.

58. Li, J., Duan, Q., Zhang, E., & Wang, J. (2018). Applications of shape memory polymers in kinetic buildings. *Advances in Materials Science and Engineering*, *2018*(1), 7453698.

59. Vakil, A. U., Ramezani, M., & Monroe, M. B. B. (2022). Magnetically actuated shape memory polymers for on-demand drug delivery. *Materials*, *15*(20), 7279.

60. Vialle, G., Di Prima, M., Hocking, E., Gall, K., Garmestani, H., Sanderson, T., & Arzberger, S. C. (2009). Remote activation of nanomagnetite reinforced shape memory polymer foam. *Smart Materials and Structures*, *18*(11), 115014.

61. Idumah, C. I., Odera, R. S., Ezeani, E. O., Low, J. H., Tanjung, F. A., Damiri, F., & Luing, W. S. (2023). Construction, characterization, properties and multifunctional applications of stimuli-responsive shape memory polymeric nanoarchitectures: A review. *Polymer-Plastics Technology and Materials*, *62*(10), 1247–1272.

62. Xiao, R., & Huang, W. M. (2020). Heating/solvent responsive shape-memory polymers for implant biomedical devices in minimally invasive surgery: Current status and challenge. *Macromolecular Bioscience*, *20*(8), 2000108.

63. Basak, S., & Bandyopadhyay, A. (2021). Solvent responsive shape memory polymers-evolution, current status, and future outlook. *Macromolecular Chemistry and Physics*, *222*(19), 2100195.

64. Chan, B. Q. Y., Heng, S. J. W., Liow, S. S., Zhang, K., & Loh, X. J. (2017). Dual-responsive hybrid thermoplastic shape memory polyurethane. *Materials Chemistry Frontiers*, *1*(4), 767–779.

65. Fang, Y., Ni, Y., Choi, B., Leo, S. Y., Gao, J., Ge, B., ... & Jiang, P. (2015). Chromogenic photonic crystals enabled by novel vapor-responsive shape-memory polymers. *Advanced Materials*, *27*(24), 3696–3704.
66. Lu, H. (2012). A simulation method to analyze chemo-mechanical behavior of swelling-induced shape-memory polymer in response to solvent. *Journal of Applied Polymer Science*, *123*(2), 1137–1146.

Why Are Solvent-Responsive Shape Memory Polymers Gaining Interest in the 21st Century?

3

Over the past two decades, shape memory polymers (SMPs) have emerged as a focal point of extensive research within the broader domain of stimulus-responsive polymers. Traditionally, heat has been the primary stimulus utilized to trigger shape recovery, owing to its convenience and widespread availability [1]. However, there are situations where accessing heat to initiate the shape memory effect (SME) poses challenges or where the use of heat may be undesirable altogether.

In such scenarios, athermal shape recovery induced by solvents or moisture emerges as an optimal alternative. This approach offers a solution when heat accessibility is limited or when avoiding heat altogether is preferable. Notably, solvent-induced SMPs have gained prominence, particularly in biomedical applications [1]. Here, the fluidic environment within the human body serves as the natural stimulus for inducing shape recovery. The application of solvent-induced SMPs holds significant promise in the biomedical field, where precise control over shape transformation in response to environmental cues is crucial. By harnessing the inherent properties of solvents present within the body, such as

 DOI: 10.1201/9781003593805-3

moisture or specific chemical compositions, these SMPs can exhibit tailored responses to achieve desired functionalities.

For instance, in medical implants or devices, solvent-induced shape recovery allows for minimally invasive procedures where heat application may not be feasible or safe. Additionally, the ability to trigger shape changes using physiological fluids enables dynamic adjustments in response to biological processes or external interventions. Overall, the utilization of solvent-induced SMPs represents a notable advancement, offering a versatile and adaptable approach to achieve athermal shape recovery. As research in this area continues to evolve, the potential applications of solvent-induced SMPs are poised to expand further, driving innovation in diverse fields ranging from biomedicine to materials science and beyond.

Solvent-responsive SMPs are capturing a growing level of interest in the scientific and industrial communities for several compelling reasons. First and foremost, their remarkable SME, where they can memorize a predetermined shape and return to it when exposed to specific solvents, presents a wide range of possibilities. This unique property has led to innovative applications that address some of today's most pressing challenges (Figure 3.1).

Figure 3.1 provides an overview of the evolution of SMPs up to the present, as compiled from SciFinder using relevant keywords. This visualization traces the trajectory of SMP development, shedding light on key milestones and trends observed in the field. The early stages of SMP development predominantly focused on thermoresponsive polymers [3–5]. Among the various stimuli utilized to trigger SMPs, thermoresponsive variants have consistently garnered attention due to their several inherent advantages. These include straightforward transition processes, precise control over thermal transition temperatures, and the manifestation of excellent SMEs [6–8].

A significant development occurred in 2005 with the introduction of light-induced SMPs. While papers in the early 2000s began exploring light-induced changes in polymer shapes, such as bending, contraction, or volume alterations, it was the pioneering work of Dr. Andreas Lendlein that catalyzed significant advancements in light-activated SMPs [8–11]. Dr. Lendlein's research marked a turning point, propelling the exploration and application of light-induced SMEs to new heights.

Overall, Figure 3.1 provides valuable insights into the dynamic landscape of SMP research, showcasing the diversification of stimuli and the emergence of novel applications over time. As the field continues to evolve, the exploration of new stimuli and the refinement of existing SMP technologies promise to unlock further opportunities for innovation and advancement.

However, the growth of solvent-responsive SMPs began primarily due to their remarkable application in self-healing materials. For instance, Bai et al. developed polymer networks that were synthesized through a straightforward

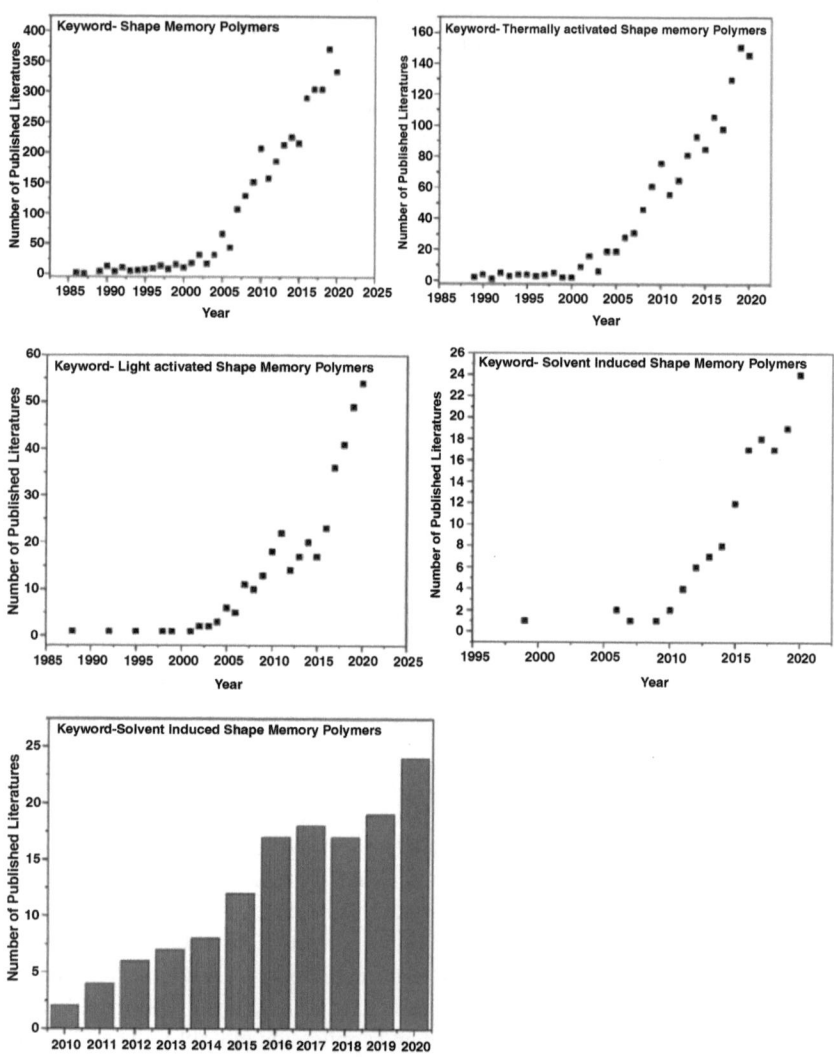

FIGURE 3.1 Evolution of the shape memory polymers in terms of published articles and the growth in the research focusing on solvent-induced SMP in the last ten years (Data extracted from SciFinder with the keywords). Reproduced with permission from [2], copyright reserved Wiley 2021.

crosslinking reaction involving poly(vinyl butyral) (PVB) and hexamethylene diisocyanate. Remarkably, these polymer networks demonstrated exceptional mechanical strength, boasting tensile modulus and tensile strength values exceeding 1 GPa and 40 MPa, respectively, at room temperature (Figure 3.2) [12]. Leveraging PVB as the switching domain, these polymer networks exhibited impressive thermal- and solvent-induced shape memory properties, achieving a remarkable R_f of 99.9% and R_r of 98.2%. Additionally, the polymer networks exhibited the ability to recover their shape when immersed in different solvents, and the speed of this recovery was contingent on both the crosslinked density and the properties of the solvents used. Furthermore, the scratch self-healing assessments illustrates that the polymer networks' ability to repeatedly mend themselves, pointing toward promising future applications for these materials (Figure 3.2) [12].

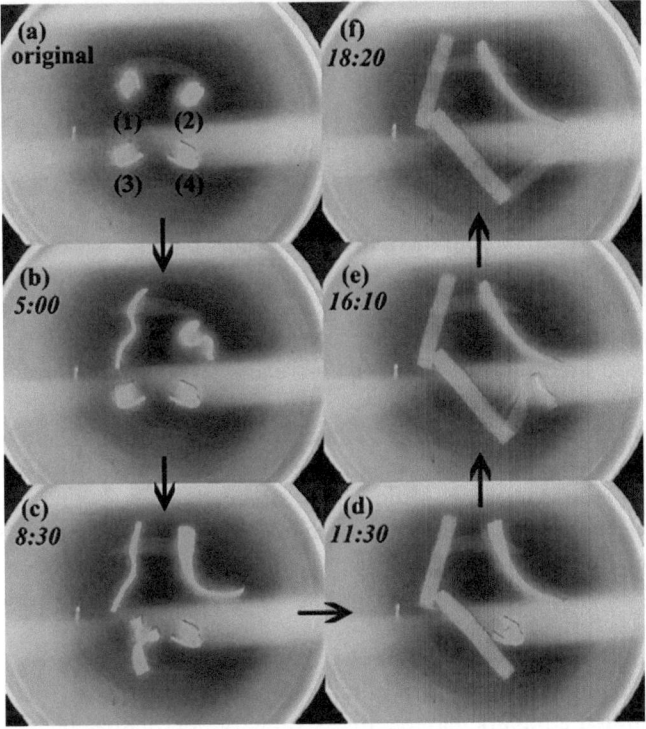

FIGURE 3.2   The shape recovery process of polymer networks that were synthesized through a straightforward crosslinking reaction involving poly(vinyl butyral) (PVB) and hexamethylene diisocyanate. Reproduced with permission from [13], copyright reserved Royal Society of Chemistry 2014.

By integrating SMPs into a wide array of products and structures, including coatings, composites, and even concrete, these materials can autonomously repair themselves when exposed to a suitable solvent. This self-healing capability holds the potential to revolutionize industries, particularly in the fields of infrastructure and manufacturing. It can lead to substantial reductions in maintenance costs, prolonged product lifespans, and enhanced overall sustainability [13,14].

In the field of smart textiles, solvent-responsive SMPs offer unprecedented versatility [15]. By integrating these polymers into fabrics, clothing, or wearables, it becomes possible to create garments that adapt to changing environmental conditions or user preferences. For example, such textiles can respond to temperature changes by altering their thermal properties, providing insulation in cold weather and breathability in warm conditions [16]. Additionally, they can find applications in medical textiles, such as bandages that adapt to wound conditions or compression garments that adjust to the wearer's needs.

Furthermore, the potential of solvent-responsive SMPs extends even further to the dynamic field of soft robotics. Within the realm of soft robotics, SMPs' unique responsiveness to solvents bestows them with the capacity to facilitate the creation of exceptionally flexible and adaptable robotic systems. These innovative robots possess the remarkable ability to undergo real-time changes in both their shape and functionality, setting the stage for a multitude of transformative applications [17]. Liang et al. have recently introduced a novel class of fully physically crosslinked hydrogels characterized by remarkable mechanical properties, including exceptional strength, toughness, stretchability, and responsiveness to solvents. These hydrogels were synthesized through a two-step manufacturing process, which involved free radical polymerization and subsequent soaking. This approach facilitated the establishment of robust physical interactions, particularly involving PAA-Fe^{3+} metal complexation and hydrogen bonding, ultimately yielding hydrogels possessing exceptional mechanical attributes (Figure 3.3) [18].

Specifically, the resulting hydrogels displayed an impressive tensile strength of approximately 5.14 MPa, signifying their exceptional resistance to deformation. Furthermore, these hydrogels exhibited an extraordinary stretchability of around 1000%, highlighting their capacity to endure substantial elongation without failure. In terms of toughness, the hydrogels demonstrated a remarkable toughness value of approximately 20.36 MJ/m^3, underscoring their ability to absorb energy and resist fracture effectively. Additionally, these hydrogels displayed excellent flexibility, with a modulus of roughly 0.53 MPa, indicating their adaptability to various applications. Notably, Liang et al.'s hydrogels also exhibited a noteworthy self-recovery property, with a self-recovery rate of 67.2% even when subjected to a strain as high as 800% (Figure 3.3) [18]. This characteristic further enhances their potential utility in diverse fields where material resilience and adaptability are crucial.

Solvent-responsive SMP-based robots have demonstrated notable utility, particularly in search and rescue missions. These environments, often characterized by disaster scenarios where conventional rigid robots may struggle, highlight the value of SMP-based robots. Their unique capability to alter their shape enables them to navigate through tight and intricate spaces, access

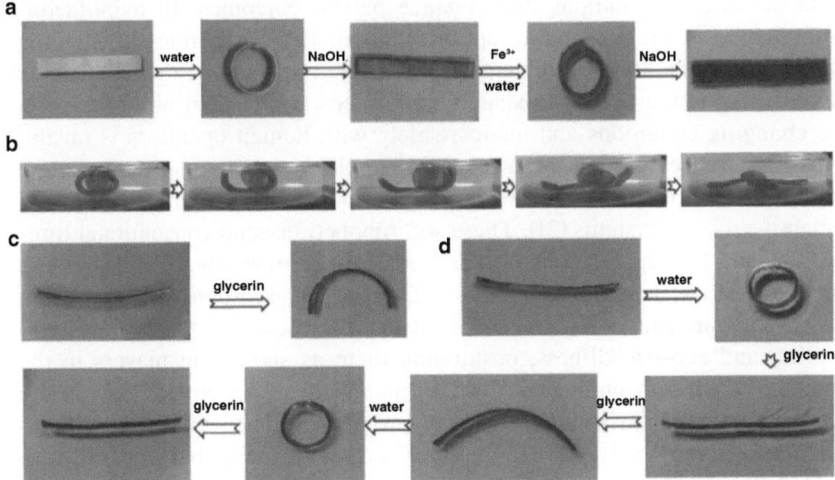

FIGURE 3.3 (a) The repeatable deformation of the hydrogel (deformable hydrogel with remarkable mechanical strength, toughness, stretchability, and solvent-responsive properties is synthesized through a two-step process. Initially, it is created via free radical polymerization carried out at room temperature. Subsequently, the hydrogel is immersed in an aqueous solution containing Fe^{3+} ions by treating with water, NaOH, and Fe^{3+} alternately. (b) The opening of hydrogel flower. (c) The deformation of the hydrogel (deformable hydrogel with remarkable mechanical strength, toughness, stretchability, and solvent-responsive properties is synthesized through a two-step process). Initially, it is created via free radical polymerization carried out at room temperature. Subsequently, the hydrogel is immersed in an aqueous solution containing Fe^{3+} ions soaking in glycerin. (d) The repeatable deformation of the hydrogel (deformable hydrogel with remarkable mechanical strength, toughness, stretchability, and solvent-responsive properties is synthesized through a two-step process). Initially, it is created via free radical polymerization carried out at room temperature. Subsequently, the hydrogel is immersed in an aqueous solution containing Fe^{3+} ions by soaking in water and glycerin alternately. Reproduced with permission from [18], copyright reserved Elsevier 2022.

confined areas, and play a crucial role in locating survivors or evaluating hazardous conditions. Their flexibility and adaptability in such contexts make them indispensable assets, providing swift and versatile responses crucial for effective rescue operations [18,19].

Additionally, we envision diverse applications for solvent-responsive SMP-based soft robots, extending beyond search and rescue missions to healthcare and manufacturing settings [20]. Their pliable and shape-shifting attributes ensure safe and seamless collaboration with humans. In healthcare, these robots can facilitate minimally invasive procedures, enabling precise and delicate interventions that enhance patient outcomes. In manufacturing, they offer the potential to optimize automation by seamlessly adapting to various tasks, thereby enhancing efficiency. Importantly, they contribute to ensuring human safety in shared workspaces, where their ability to react to changing conditions and interact safely with human operators is invaluable. We foresee solvent-responsive SMPs holding immense promise in the realm of soft robotics, empowering the development of highly flexible and adaptive robotic systems [21]. These soft robots transcend conventional limitations and find applications in search and rescue missions, healthcare, and manufacturing, ushering in a new era of versatile and responsive automation.

SMPs are increasingly recognized for their potential to drive sustainability and eco-friendliness, positioning them as significant players in the realm of environmentally conscious technological advancements [22]. A key attribute that sets SMPs apart in this regard is their ability to utilize environmentally friendly solvents, aligning perfectly with the global imperative to adopt green technologies and materials for a more sustainable future.

The utilization of environmentally friendly solvents alongside SMPs offers several advantages that resonate with the broader environmental agenda [23]. Firstly, it diminishes reliance on and consumption of harmful or non-renewable resources, promoting resource conservation. This conservation not only upholds the principles of sustainable development but also helps mitigate the depletion of critical resources, often linked with adverse environmental impacts.

Furthermore, the compatibility of SMPs with environmentally friendly solvents facilitates a reduction in hazardous waste production and emissions. This holds significance as many conventional materials and processes generate pollutants and wastes that pose environmental threats. By opting for eco-friendly solvents alongside SMPs, industries can mitigate their ecological footprint and minimize their contribution to pollution, thereby making positive strides toward environmental preservation [22].

The incorporation of SMPs into various applications, driven by the use of sustainable solvents, exemplifies a broader trend toward green and clean technologies. This trend is being championed globally as part of efforts to combat climate change and reduce the environmental degradation associated with industrial and technological activities. Consequently, SMPs have emerged as a favorable choice for researchers, engineers, and industries that seek to align their operations with sustainability goals, reduce carbon footprints, and adhere to eco-friendly practices [24]. The synergy between SMPs and environmentally friendly solvents not only enhances the materials' appeal but also positions them as promising contributors to the ongoing global endeavor to promote green technologies and sustainable materials. This alignment with sustainability objectives underscores the potential of SMPs to drive positive change in various industries, fostering a more eco-conscious and environmentally responsible future.

The burgeoning interest in solvent-responsive SMPs is a result of their exceptional combination of shape memory properties and solvent responsiveness. Their applications are multifaceted, spanning self-healing materials, smart textiles, soft robotics, and sustainable technology solutions. As research and innovation continue to advance in the realm of SMPs, the transformative potential of these materials remains vast and largely untapped. Their unique properties offer a wealth of opportunities for novel applications, and their versatility ensures that they will continue to be a subject of intense exploration and development in the coming years. The current surge of interest in SMPs is a testament to their capacity to revolutionize industries and technologies, and as scientists, engineers, and innovators delve deeper into the possibilities they offer, we can anticipate even more groundbreaking applications and solutions to emerge. The journey of solvent-responsive SMPs is far from over, and its evolution promises to shape a more adaptive, sustainable, and technologically advanced future.

REFERENCES

1. Xiao, R., & Huang, W. M. (2020). Heating/solvent responsive shape-memory polymers for implant biomedical devices in minimally invasive surgery: Current status and challenge. *Macromolecular Bioscience*, 20(8), 2000108.
2. Basak, S., & Bandyopadhyay, A. (2021). Solvent responsive shape memory polymers-evolution, current status, and future outlook. *Macromolecular Chemistry and Physics*, 222(19), 2100195.
3. Chan, B. Q. Y., Heng, S. J. W., Liow, S. S., Zhang, K., & Loh, X. J. (2017). Dual-responsive hybrid thermoplastic shape memory polyurethane. *Materials Chemistry Frontiers*, 1(4), 767–779.
4. Fang, Y., Ni, Y., Choi, B., Leo, S. Y., Gao, J., Ge, B., ... & Jiang, P. (2015). Chromogenic photonic crystals enabled by novel vapor-responsive shape-memory polymers. *Advanced Materials*, 27(24), 3696–3704.

5. Lu, H. (2012). A simulation method to analyze chemo-mechanical behavior of swelling-induced shape-memory polymer in response to solvent. *Journal of Applied Polymer Science*, *123*(2), 1137–1146.

6. Basak, S., & Bandyopadhyay, A. (2022). Two-way semicrystalline shape memory elastomers: Development and current research trends. *Advanced Engineering Materials*, *24*(10), 2200257.

7. Kong, D., Li, J., Guo, A., Zhang, X., & Xiao, X. (2019). Self-healing high temperature shape memory polymer. *European Polymer Journal*, *120*, 109279.

8. Fulcher, J. T., Lu, Y. C., Tandon, G. P., & Foster, D. C. (2010). Thermomechanical characterization of shape memory polymers using high temperature nanoindentation. *Polymer Testing*, *29*(5), 544–552.

9. Behl, M., Razzaq, M. Y., & Lendlein, A. (2010). Multifunctional shape-memory polymers. *Advanced Materials*, *22*(31), 3388–3410.

10. Lendlein, A., Jiang, H., Jünger, O., & Langer, R. (2005). Light-induced shape-memory polymers. *Nature*, *434*(7035), 879–882.

11. Lendlein, A., & Gould, O. E. (2019). Reprogrammable recovery and actuation behaviour of shape-memory polymers. *Nature Reviews Materials*, *4*(2), 116–133.

12. Camacho-Lopez, M., Finkelmann, H., Palffy-Muhoray, P., & Shelley, M. (2004). Fast liquid-crystal elastomer swims into the dark. *Nature Materials*, *3*(5), 307–310.

13. Bai, Y., Chen, Y., Wang, Q., & Wang, T. (2014). Poly (vinyl butyral) based polymer networks with dual-responsive shape memory and self-healing properties. *Journal of Materials Chemistry A*, *2*(24), 9169–9177.

14. Neuser, S., Michaud, V., & White, S. R. (2012). Improving solvent-based self-healing materials through shape memory alloys. *Polymer*, *53*(2), 370–378.

15. Lu, C., Liu, Y., Liu, X., Wang, C., Wang, J., & Chu, F. (2018). Sustainable multiple-and multistimulus-shape-memory and self-healing elastomers with semi-interpenetrating network derived from biomass via bulk radical polymerization. *ACS Sustainable Chemistry & Engineering*, *6*(5), 6527–6535.

16. Xiao, X., Hu, J., Gui, X., & Qian, K. (2017). Shape memory investigation of α-keratin fibers as multi-coupled stimuli of responsive smart materials. *Polymers*, *9*(3), 87.

17. Thakur, S. (2017). Shape memory polymers for smart textile applications. Bipin Kumar (Ed.), In *Textiles for advanced applications* (pp. 323–336), Hong Kong Polytechnic University, China: Intechopen.

18. Liang, Y., Shen, Y., & Liang, H. (2022). Solvent-responsive strong hydrogel with programmable deformation and reversible shape memory for load-carrying soft robot. *Materials Today Communications*, *30*, 103067.

19. Li, G., Gao, T., Fan, G., Liu, Z., Liu, Z., Jiang, J., & Zhao, Y. (2019). Photoresponsive shape memory hydrogels for complex deformation and solvent-driven actuation. *ACS Applied Materials & Interfaces*, *12*(5), 6407–6418.

20. Patadiya, J., Gawande, A., Joshi, G., & Kandasubramanian, B. (2021). Additive manufacturing of shape memory polymer composites for futuristic technology. *Industrial & Engineering Chemistry Research*, *60*(44), 15885–15912.

21. Shi, S., Cui, M., Sun, F., Zhu, K., Iqbal, M. I., Chen, X., ... & Hu, J. (2021). An innovative solvent-responsive coiling–expanding stent. Advanced Materials, 33(32), 2101005.

22. Toncheva, A., Khelifa, F., Paint, Y., Voué, M., Lambert, P., Dubois, P., & Raquez, J. M. (2018). Fast IR-actuated shape-memory polymers using in situ silver nanoparticle-grafted cellulose nanocrystals. *ACS Applied Materials & Interfaces*, *10*(35), 29933–29942.

23. Musarurwa, H., & Tavengwa, N. T. (2022). Recyclable polysaccharide/stimuli-responsive polymer composites and their applications in water remediation. *Carbohydrate Polymers*, *298*, 120083.

24. Alauzen, T., Ross, S., & Madbouly, S. (2021). Biodegradable shape-memory polymers and composites. *Physical Sciences Reviews*, *8*(9), 2049–2070.

Effect of Solvent Diffusion on the Shape Memory Process and Shape Memory Efficacy of a Solvent-Excited Shape Memory Polymer

4

4.1 FACTORS INFLUENCING SOLVENT ABSORPTION IN POLYMERS

The capacity of a polymer to absorb solvents is a crucial aspect that lies at the heart of the fascinating phenomenon of solvent- and moisture-triggered shape memory effects [1,2]. This property is deeply rooted in the polymer's

DOI: 10.1201/9781003593805-4

chemical composition, molecular structure, and the intricate intermolecular interactions within its matrix [1]. Collectively, these factors determine the polymer's capability to effectively interact with and absorb solvents.

This interaction is far from passive; it represents an active engagement that plays a central role in shaping the material's responsiveness and its remarkable ability to revert to its original form when stimulated by solvents or moisture [3]. The polymer's capacity to absorb solvents is thus a dynamic process that drives its shape memory behavior, underscoring the intricate relationship between molecular-level interactions and macroscopic material properties.

Central to this phenomenon is the polymer's innate capacity to absorb solvents to varying degrees. Polymers exhibit a wide spectrum of solvent affinity, ranging from minimal absorption to an impressive ability to soak up several times their original weight in solvents. This variation in solvent absorption reflects the unique molecular composition of each polymer.

Several factors influence a polymer's propensity to absorb solvents. The presence of specific functional groups within the polymer's structure is key as these groups can form chemical bonds with solvent molecules. Additionally, the arrangement and configuration of the polymer chains play a crucial role in determining how readily solvent molecules can permeate the material. Moreover, the type of intermolecular bonds present within the polymer matrix also affects its overall receptivity to solvents. Weak intermolecular forces may allow solvents to penetrate the polymer more easily, leading to increased absorption.

Thus, the extent to which a polymer absorbs solvents is governed by a complex interplay of its molecular characteristics, including the presence of functional groups, chain structure, and intermolecular bonds. These factors collectively dictate the material's interaction with solvents and shape its behavior in solvent-induced processes such as shape memory effects.

4.2 QUANTITATIVE ANALYSIS: THE VRENTAS/DUDA FREE-VOLUME DIFFUSION MODEL

From a quantitative perspective, the Vrentas/Duda free-volume diffusion model stands as an impressive and reliable tool in the realm of polymer science [4–6]. It has demonstrated its exceptional ability to precisely correlate diffusion coefficients of polymers and solvents across expansive spectrums of concentration and temperature [4]. This model represents a noteworthy milestone in our understanding of how polymer-solvent interactions manifest and evolve under varying conditions. At its core, this model offers a systematic approach to deciphering the intricate amalgamation of molecules within a polymer matrix as they engage with and traverse through the solvent molecules. It achieves this by tapping into the concept of free volume, a concept rooted in the spaces between polymer chains and molecules. These interstitial regions, known as free volume, serve as the highways through which solvent molecules navigate as they move within the polymer structure. The model's success lies in its adeptness at capturing the nuances of how diffusion coefficients change as a function of concentration and temperature. It offers a quantitative framework that allows researchers to predict, with remarkable accuracy, how fast molecules will move through a given polymer-solvent system under different circumstances. This predictive power is indispensable in various scientific and industrial applications, particularly in fields such as materials science, chemical engineering, and polymer processing [4–6].

In the free-volume theory of Vrentas and Duda [4–6], the expression for the binary mutual diffusion coefficient D can be written as

$$D = \frac{D_1 \rho_2 V_2 \rho_1}{RT} \frac{\delta \mu_1}{(\delta \rho_1)} T, P \tag{4.1}$$

where

$$D_1 = D_{01} \exp\left[-\frac{\gamma(\omega_1 V_1 + \omega_2 \zeta V_2)}{V_{FH}} \right] \tag{4.2}$$

where μ_1 (solvent chemical potential) and V_{FH} (partial specific volumes of polymer and solvent) can be computed using the thermodynamic theory of Flory (1970) [7].

4.3 APPLICATIONS AND MECHANISMS OF SOLVENT-INDUCED SHAPE MEMORY EFFECTS

A comprehensive understanding of the Vrentas/Duda free-volume diffusion model and its applicability to shape memory polymers (SMPs) is elaborated upon in [4]. This model represents a powerful tool for analyzing the intricate relationship between polymer-solvent interactions and the resulting solvent responsiveness observed in SMPs. What is particularly intriguing about this model is that it highlights the multi-dimensional nature of solvent responsiveness; it isn't solely determined by a single parameter but rather a combination of several key factors. One of the central elements considered in this model is the concept of solvent chemical potential. This parameter reflects the thermodynamic driving force that compels solvent molecules to migrate within the polymer matrix. It plays a crucial role in dictating the rate and extent of solvent diffusion, which directly impacts the shape memory effect in SMPs. The interplay between the chemical potential and the polymer-solvent system's characteristics is a critical aspect of understanding and predicting the behavior of these smart materials.

Moreover, the model considers the partial specific volumes of both the polymer and the solvent. These values capture the spatial requirements of individual polymer chains and solvent molecules within the system. The intermolecular spaces, or free volume, available for solvent molecules to traverse through are influenced by these specific volumes. This factor is pivotal in determining how easily solvents can permeate the polymer structure and, consequently, how quickly the shape memory effect can be initiated and controlled. The Flory-Huggins interaction parameter [8], another key component, quantifies the affinity between the polymer and the solvent. This parameter captures the thermodynamic compatibility of the two entities. A favorable interaction parameter implies a strong attraction between the polymer and the solvent, facilitating solvent uptake and, consequently, shape memory response. Conversely, an unfavorable parameter suggests repulsion, which can impede solvent diffusion and affect the shape memory behavior accordingly. Temperature also emerges as a critical variable. It influences the mobility of molecules within the polymer-solvent system. Changes in temperature can lead to alterations in the diffusion rates and, consequently, affect the kinetics of shape memory responses. This temperature sensitivity is crucial to consider when designing SMPs for applications where temperature fluctuations are significant [7].

It's worth noting that evaluating the parameters of this theory typically requires a combination of readily available data, such as density and viscosity information, along with a relatively small amount of equilibrium and diffusivity data. This makes the model not only theoretically sound but also practically feasible for researchers and engineers working with SMPs. This combination of accessible data and predictive power empowers scientists to better understand and manipulate the solvent responsiveness of SMPs.

The Vrentas/Duda free-volume diffusion model represents a comprehensive approach to understanding the multifaceted nature of solvent responsiveness in SMPs. By taking into account factors like solvent chemical potential, specific volumes, interaction parameters, and temperature, this model provides a holistic framework for predicting and optimizing the behavior of these remarkable materials. It is a valuable tool for researchers and engineers seeking to harness the full potential of SMPs in diverse applications from biomedical devices to smart textiles and beyond [7,8].

When a polymer exhibits a pronounced affinity for solvents, it demonstrates an inherent capacity to absorb significant quantities of these liquid substances. This absorption capability is not to be underestimated as it can vary widely, ranging from a few modest percentage points to a truly astonishing several hundred percentage points of the polymer's initial weight.

This extraordinary property serves as the cornerstone for the polymer's metamorphosis into a dynamic and highly responsive material, replete with the potential for remarkable transformations. The degree to which solvents are absorbed indeed stands as a pivotal determinant in shaping the material's overall responsiveness and behavior. As the polymer absorbs solvents, it undergoes substantial dimensional changes, manifested as noticeable swelling due to the influx of these foreign substances. This swelling, in essence, serves as the catalyst for the material's remarkable shape memory effect. It enables the polymer to transiently assume a novel form, adapting to the environmental stimulus provided by the solvent.

This process of swelling and shape adaptation underscores the polymer's remarkable versatility and adaptability, making it suitable for a wide array of applications across various industries. From biomedical devices to smart materials, the ability of these polymers to respond dynamically to their surroundings holds immense promise for innovation and advancement in numerous fields.

Importantly, when the external solvent stimulus is eventually withdrawn or reduced, the polymer, drawing upon its intrinsic memory, undergoes a gradual yet precise reversion to its original shape. This phase of the process unfolds with a notable degree of reliability, marking one of the defining characteristics of shape memory materials.

The capacity of a polymer to imbibe solvents in significant quantities opens the gateway to a dynamic interplay between the material and its environment. It is this interaction that lies at the core of the shape memory phenomenon observed in polymers. The polymer's ability to absorb, swell, and subsequently recover its original configuration showcases the versatility and potential of these materials across a spectrum of applications, from biomedical devices to smart materials in engineering and beyond. The ability of a polymer to absorb solvents to varying degrees represents a pivotal feature in shaping its responsiveness and its capacity to undergo remarkable transformations. This phenomenon underscores the multifaceted nature of polymers and their dynamic interactions with the surrounding environment, offering a wealth of possibilities for innovative applications across diverse scientific and industrial domains.

Measurement techniques are essential for evaluating the behavior of these polymers in response to solvents. Researchers often employ the swelling ratio as a primary measurement. This method involves immersing the polymer in a solvent or subjecting it to moisture and tracking dimensional changes over time. The swelling ratio is calculated by dividing the final swollen dimensions by the original dimensions. This approach provides valuable data on how a polymer interacts with different solvents or moisture levels.

For instance, Li et al. developed a sulfobetaine methacrylate (SBMA) copolymerized with 2,3-dihydroxypropyl methacrylate (DHMA) in the presence of boric acid as a crosslinking agent, generating a novel thermo- and moisture-responsive zwitterionic SMP [2]. Through the assessment of swelling ratios under different relative humidity conditions, a clear and direct relationship emerged between the equilibrium swelling ratio and the levels of relative humidity. This investigation underscored the crucial role played by solvent absorption in the realization of shape memory effects. Figure 4.1c shows the water absorption capacity of these zwitterionic SMPs, and the rate of water absorption increases with an increase in relative humidity. Similarly, Figure 4.1b illustrates the contraction (shape memory property) of these zwitterionic SMPs, and it correlates directly to the water absorbed as more the water absorbed, higher will be the contraction, the same as predicted by the Vrentas/Duda free-volume diffusion model [2].

One noteworthy research endeavor, led by Li et al. in 2019, delved into the development of copolymers that exhibit a remarkable sensitivity to water. Their work, documented in two separate studies [1,2], shed light on the potential of these water-responsive copolymers. These materials are designed to undergo significant changes in their shape and properties in the presence of water, making them particularly suitable for applications in fields such as biomedicine, environmental sensing, and controlled drug release.

In another innovative study by Liu et al. in 2015, a thermoresponsive and water-responsive shape memory polymer nanocomposite network was developed through the chemical crosslinking of cellulose nanocrystals (CNCs) with polycaprolactone (PCL) and polyethylene glycol (PEG). The nanocomposite network underwent a comprehensive characterization process, encompassing the analysis of its microstructure, crosslink density, water contact angle, water uptake capacity, crystallinity, thermal behavior, and static as well as dynamic mechanical properties. The investigation yielded noteworthy results, indicating that the PEG–PCL–CNC nanocomposite exhibited remarkable shape memory effects when exposed to variations in temperature and immersion in water, particularly when submerged in an aqueous environment at 37°C, mimicking physiological conditions (Figure 4.2) [9].

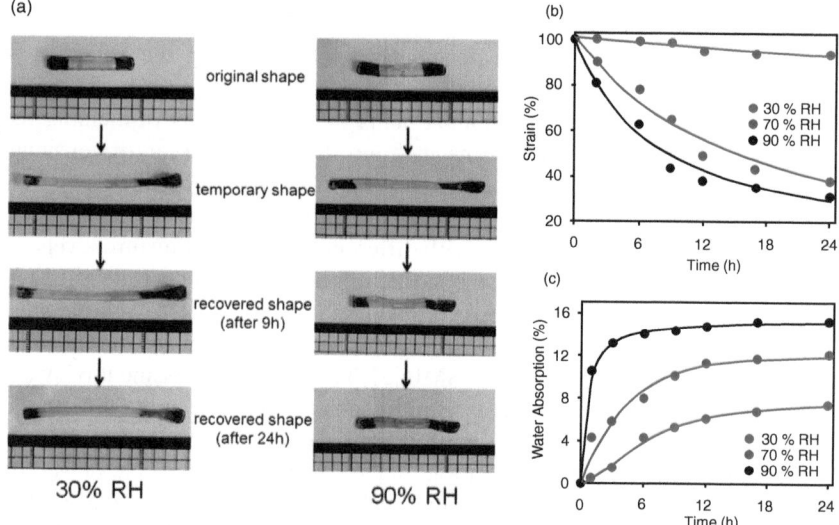

FIGURE 4.1   (a) Images illustrating the shape memory transformation of the zwitterionic shape memory polymer triggered by the absorption of moisture, either from the ambient air (at 30% relative humidity) or within a controlled environmental chamber (at 90% relative humidity). (b) The contraction of the zwitterionic shape memory polymer, induced by moisture, while it retains elongated temporary shapes under varying environmental humidity conditions. (c) Examination of the water absorption characteristics of the zwitterionic shape memory polymer under diverse environmental humidity levels. Reproduced with permission from [2], copyright reserved Wiley 2019.

The introduction of CNCs into the blend of PEG and PCL, both of which possessed relatively low molecular weights, notably augmented the mechanical properties of the resulting nanocomposite. This enhancement enhances the material's potential utility in a variety of fields, including healthcare and engineering. Additionally, the nanocomposites demonstrated promising cytocompatibility through Alamar Blue assays involving osteoblasts, signifying their compatibility with biological systems. This observation highlights the potential of these nanocomposites as smart biomaterials for various biomedical applications (Figure 4.2) [9].

The significance of solvent diversity and its corresponding behavior plays a pivotal role in the comprehensive understanding of shape memory effects within polymer systems. While water remains a frequently employed solvent due to its ubiquity and inherent safety, it is crucial to acknowledge that organic solvents also possess the capability to elicit shape memory responses

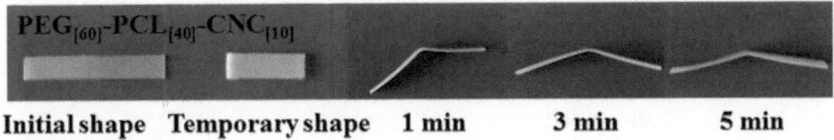

FIGURE 4.2 Demonstrating the water-responsive shape memory process of PEG–PCL–CNC nanocomposites in 37 °C water. Reproduced with permission from [9], copyright reserved American Chemical Society 2015.

in polymers. A noteworthy study conducted by Xiao et al. in 2015 illuminated the intriguing parallel between the absorption behavior of organic solvents and that of water within a polymer matrix (Figure 4.3) [10].

Xiao et al.'s research findings shed light on an intriguing aspect of polymer behavior: the similarity in absorption characteristics between organic solvents and water when interacting with polymers. This discovery emphasizes the remarkable versatility of polymers as they demonstrate the ability to respond not only to aqueous environments but also to a diverse range of organic solvents. Such versatility significantly broadens the scope of potential applications for shape memory materials, extending their utility beyond traditional aqueous settings [10].

However, amidst this exciting revelation, an essential caveat emerges: the diffusion rate and extent of swelling can vary significantly depending on the specific combination of polymer and solvent. This variability underscores the complexity of polymer-solvent interactions and highlights the need for careful consideration when designing and implementing shape memory materials for practical applications. Researchers and engineers must account for these nuances to ensure optimal performance and reliability in diverse environments.

Undoubtedly, the kinetics of diffusion and the extent of swelling are intricately linked to the specific pairing of polymer and solvent. The variations witnessed in these parameters underscore the paramount importance of a judiciously chosen solvent for a given application. The customized selection of solvent stands as a pivotal factor, serving not only to guarantee the attainment of the desired shape memory response but also to meticulously fine-tune the overall performance and functionality of polymer-based materials. The contemplation of solvent diversity and its inherent behavior emerges as an elemental facet when delving into the realm of shape memory effects within polymers. The adaptability of polymers in their responsiveness to both aqueous and organic solvents presents a vast array of opportunities across diverse applications. Nevertheless, the prudent and deliberate selection of the most fitting solvent remains an indispensable determinant in realizing the targeted

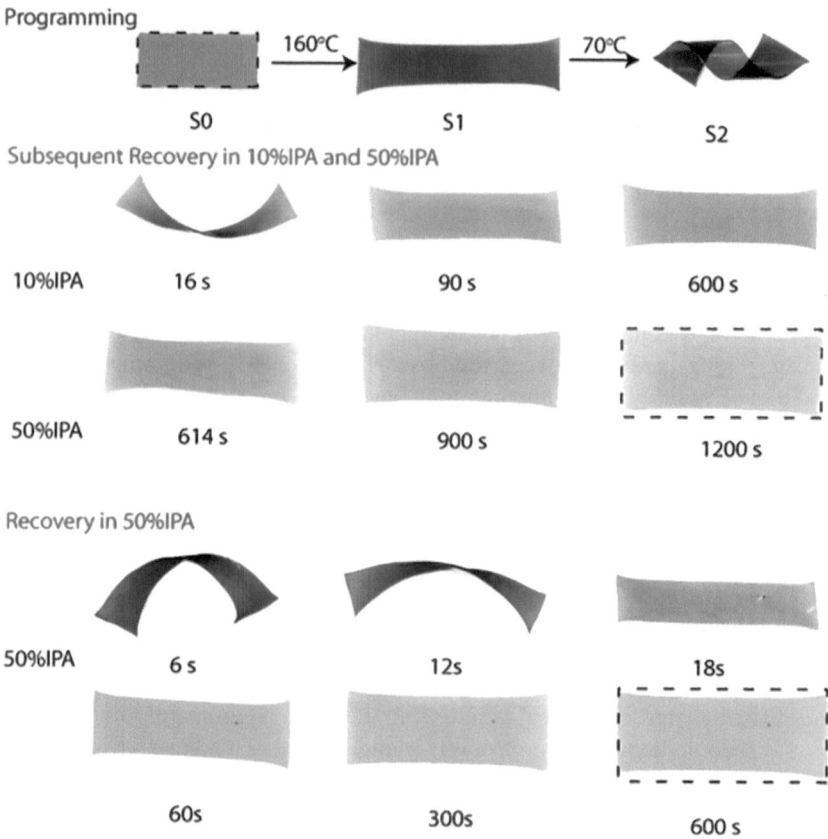

FIGURE 4.3   Shape recovery demonstration of Nafion films programmed with two temporary shapes at 160 °C and 70 °C, recovered successively in 10% IPA and 50% IPA and recovered in 50% IPA. Reproduced with permission from [10], copyright reserved Royal Society of Chemistry 2015.

shape memory characteristics and in optimizing the overall efficacy of these materials across an array of contexts and industries [9,10].

Circumscribing on the swelling methodology, swelling tests are commonly used in materials science to study how a material interacts with a solvent. These tests involve immersing a material in a solvent and observing how it absorbs the solvent over time. The amount of solvent absorbed by the material provides valuable information about its swelling behavior and can be used to determine properties such as swelling ratio, diffusion coefficient, and sorption kinetics [11].

However, while swelling tests offer insights into a material's overall solvent absorption capacity, they have limitations in providing detailed information about the distribution of solvent concentration within the material. This limitation becomes significant when dealing with materials of complex geometries or specific structural features [12]. In practice, when a material is exposed to a solvent, the concentration of the solvent near the material's surface tends to be higher than the interior. This is due to the initial contact between the material and the solvent, where the solvent molecules have easier access to the surface. As a result, the material's surface regions absorb solvent more rapidly and may undergo swelling and shape recovery before the interior regions. This phenomenon leads to gradients in solvent concentration within the material [11,12].

These concentration gradients can have a profound impact on the material's behavior. For materials with specific slender geometries or intricate structures, the uneven distribution of solvent concentration can result in unique deformation patterns. Some regions of the material may expand or contract more rapidly than others, leading to non-uniform swelling or shape changes [13,14].

Understanding these localized concentration gradients and their effects on materials is crucial for designing and engineering materials for specific applications. Researchers and engineers need to consider not only the overall swelling behavior of a material but also how solvent concentration varies within it. This knowledge can help in optimizing material properties, predicting performance, and avoiding unwanted deformations or failures in real-world applications [14].

Diffusion mechanisms can vary based on temperature and material properties. For instance, Zhao et al. conducted a study measuring the movement of the penetration front of ethanol in poly(methyl methacrylate) (PMMA) [15]. The paper explores the buckling behavior of PMMA when subjected to stimulus-responsive shape recovery processes. It investigates how PMMA, a common polymer, deforms and recovers its shape in response to external stimuli. Figure 4.4 provides an illustration of the buckling mechanism observed in pre-stretched PMMA when it is immersed in room-temperature ethanol. PMMA belongs to the category of amorphous polymers. From a thermodynamic perspective, in its stable state, PMMA exhibits a disordered, randomly coiled, and intricately entangled configuration of molecular chains (Figure 4.4).

Upon subjecting PMMA to stretching at elevated temperatures, these molecular chains undergo a rearrangement, resulting in an unstable state (Figures 4.4 and 4.5). This rearrangement leads to the localized storage of elastic energy (as indicated in previous research). Following this, upon cooling back to room temperature and unloading, there is a limited and immediate recovery (Figure 4.5). It is noteworthy that PMMA has the capacity to absorb ethanol, which subsequently softens the material through a plasticization process, as previously documented [15].

During the softening process, a gradual release of stored elastic energy occurs, starting from the outer layers and progressing inward. This release is facilitated by the recoiling and re-entanglement of the molecular chains within the material. As a result, compressive stress is generated within the softened region, as depicted in Figures 4.4 and 4.5.

In instances where the compressive force exceeds a critical threshold, it can induce buckling of the material. This phenomenon highlights the delicate balance between the applied forces and the material's structural integrity. As the softening process continues, more molecular chains undergo this transformation, leading to a progressive restoration of the material's original shape, as illustrated in Figure 4.5.

These observations corroborate previous research findings in the field, reaffirming the fundamental principles underlying the behavior of materials undergoing softening and subsequent recovery processes [15]. Understanding these mechanisms is crucial for designing and engineering materials with tailored properties and performance characteristics, with implications spanning various industries, from structural engineering to biomedical applications.

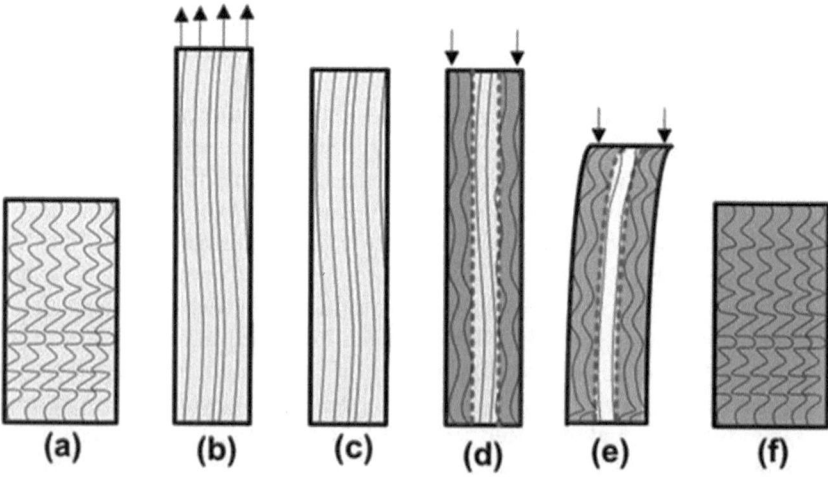

(a)   **(b)**   **(c)**   **(d)**   **(e)**   **(f)**

FIGURE 4.4   An example of the underlying mechanism. Initial amorphous PMMA, uniaxial stretching at high temperatures, cooling and unloading, penetration of ethanol and softening of the outer layer, buckling at a crucial penetration depth, and final shape upon recovery. With ethanol is the shaded area. Reproduced with permission from [15], copyright reserved AIP Publishing 2011.

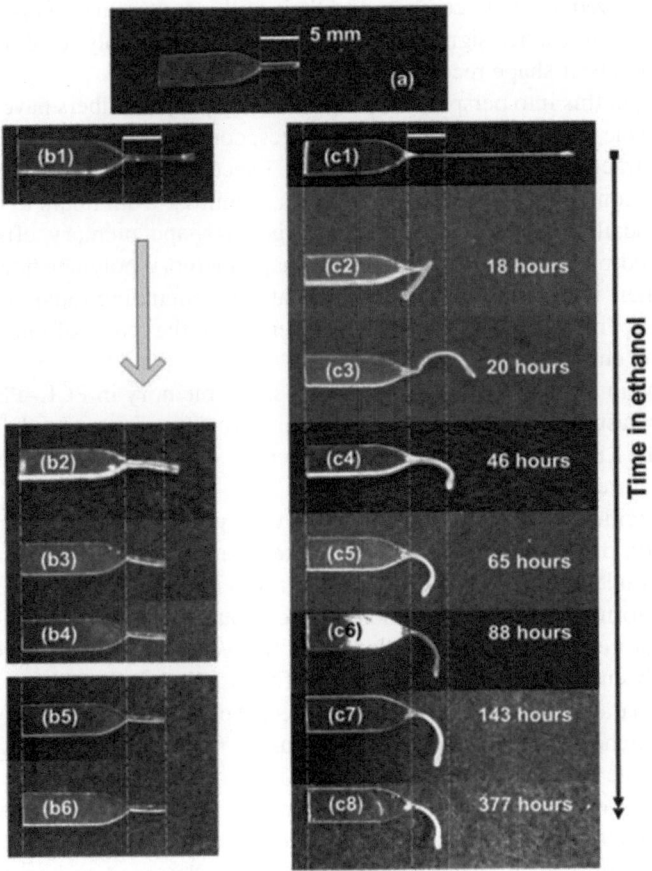

FIGURE 4.5   Recovery of PMMA upon immersing into room temperature ethanol. Reproduced with permission from [15], copyright reserved AIP Publishing 2011.

It is worth noting that this study showed that the penetration depth had a linear relationship with time, indicative of case II diffusion behavior, where polymers with glass transition temperatures (Tg) significantly higher than room temperature exhibit viscoelastic relaxation as the dominant diffusion mechanism [15,16].

Besides considering the chemical composition of polymer specimens, it's essential to acknowledge the impact of their morphology on diffusion rates. A notable study by Gu and Mather in 2013 shed light on this aspect, revealing that polymer diffusion rates experience a significant increase when materials are structured as fibers compared to their bulk counterparts. This enhanced diffusion rate carries significant implications, most notably resulting in considerably faster shape recovery times [17].

To put this into perspective, shape memory polymer fibers have achieved remarkable feats in terms of recovery times, condensing the entire process to a mere fraction of time, typically around 1 second. This achievement stands in stark contrast to the protracted periods, spanning from hours to days, that are typically observed in moisture-triggered shape memory effects. The expedited recovery times observed in shape memory polymer fibers underscore their immense potential for applications demanding rapid and precise responses, marking a substantial advancement in the realm of materials science and engineering [17].

The investigation of water-triggered shape memory in PCL–PEG-based thermoplastic polyurethanes involved subjecting specimens to deformation using the Linkam tensile tester under carefully controlled conditions at room temperature.

Specifically, the wet film and wet web were stretched to achieve an extension of up to 485% using the Linkam tensile tester and then fixed at this strain level. This fixation process involved maintaining the specimens in their deformed state for a duration of three hours, all while at ambient room temperature. This time frame allowed for the wet samples to undergo drying, crucially enabling the recrystallization of the PEG phase.

In parallel, for comparative purposes, the dry film and dry web were also stretched to a strain level of 485% using the same equipment and held at this state for a period of three hours. This duration was allocated to facilitate stress relaxation within the dry samples. Subsequently, the strain was released until the stress reached zero, as depicted in Figure 4.6. This experimental setup and procedure were meticulously designed to investigate the

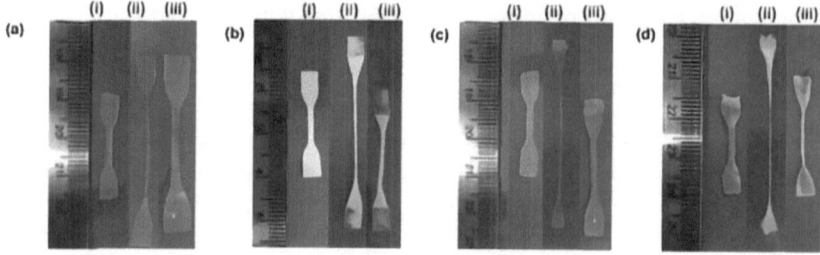

FIGURE 4.6   Wet film, wet web, dry film, and dry web form memory tests using water triggers. Original dogbone samples, Linkam-stretched and -fixed samples, and samples after stretching, fixing, and water recovery at room temperature (S/F/R) are the three types of samples. Reproduced with permission from [17], copyright reserved Royal Society of Chemistry 2013.

effect of water-triggered shape memory in PCL–PEG thermoplastic polyurethanes under controlled conditions.

Notably, through the process of fixing, which hinges on PEG recrystallization, both hydrogel samples exhibited notably higher fixing ratios (89% for the wet film and 91% for the wet web) than their dry counterparts (77% for the dry film and 70% for the dry web). Further examination of the fixing capacity of the wet samples involved the variation of fixing (drying) time. Intriguingly, it was observed that a duration of 1.5 hours was sufficiently long to attain fixing ratios as high as those achieved over a span of 3 hours. Subsequently, the highly deformed specimens were immersed in water at room temperature for a duration of ten minutes, effectively triggering the process of shape recovery. Figure 4.6 provides a visual representation, offering a comparative view of the original dogbone samples, samples subjected to stretching and fixing (abbreviated as "S/F"), and samples post-stretching, fixing, and water-induced recovery (abbreviated as "S/F/R") [17].

For the dry film, partial recovery was attained, yielding an Rr value of 44%. Interestingly, the recovery ratio of the dry web displayed a substantial increase, reaching 64% in contrast to the dry film. This divergence can be attributed to the larger surface expansion exhibited by the bulk film when submerged in water, ultimately influencing its recovery ratio to be lower. Intriguingly, by programming the specimens in their hydrogel state, their recovery ratios witnessed significant enhancement, reaching 73% for the film and an impressive 83% for the web. A plausible hypothesis suggests that for the wet samples, the PCL phase experienced limited deformation, or potentially no deformation at all, during the tensile deformation process. This hypothesis substantiates the superior recovery observed in the wet samples [17].

While discussing solvent-responsive SMPs, the mechanism of molecular sorption generally hinges on the attractive interaction between polymer chains and the penetrant. However, notable exceptions exist, such as PTFE, which repels water despite its high porosity. The nature of this interaction is intricately linked to the arrangement of functional groups, with dispersive forces playing a significant role.

When dissimilar molecules come into play, weaker intermolecular forces often give rise to a phenomenon termed void filling. In this scenario, penetrant molecules exhibit a greater affinity for each other than for the functional groups of the polymer. This challenges the conventional understanding based on the concentration gradient principle, which typically governs solvent diffusion within polymers. The attainment of thermodynamic equilibrium becomes evident when a uniform concentration is observed throughout the penetrated region, even after the penetrant supply has ceased. This indicates that the forces driving equilibrium solubility outweigh those attempting to minimize the concentration gradient, which is one of the key driving forces for shape recovery with solvents [18, 19].

Despite the theoretical framework, the measurement of concentration profiles at the diffusion front presents certain challenges. Factors such as spatial resolution and the non-uniformity of the polymer matrix can lead to broader front transitions, complicating the interpretation of experimental data [20]. These challenges underscore the complexity inherent in understanding the intricacies of solvent diffusion within polymer matrices and highlight the ongoing need for refined experimental techniques and theoretical models in this field.

The dependence of diffusion distance on $t^{1/2}$ implies that the rate of diffusion is governed by resistance to flow. This resistance is influenced by factors such as the viscosity of the penetrant, the size of the open pores, the distance from the polymer surface, and the attractive forces within the matrix, all of which determines the efficacy of the shape fixation and shape recovery of the solvent-triggered SMP [21–23].

It may be possible in future research to predict values for diffusion, solubility, and permeability by considering these factors comprehensively.

Looking ahead, the field of solvent-responsive SMPs holds immense promise for further advancements. Researchers continue to investigate diffusion mechanisms, enabling a deeper understanding of the fundamental science behind these materials. Tailoring the chemical composition, morphology, and responsiveness of these materials offers opportunities for diverse applications in biomedicine, sensors, and actuators. Optimizing solvent-triggered shape recovery in various forms, such as foams or fibers, may unlock innovative solutions across multiple industries. In conclusion, the study of solvent-responsive SMPs is multifaceted, and an ongoing research in this field offers the potential for groundbreaking developments in materials science and engineering.

REFERENCES

1. Li, A., Challapalli, A., & Li, G. (2019). 4D printing of recyclable lightweight architectures using high recovery stress shape memory polymer. *Scientific Reports, 9*(1), 7621.
2. Li, G., Wang, Y., Wang, S., Liu, Z., Liu, Z., & Jiang, J. (2019). A thermo-and moisture-responsive zwitterionic shape memory polymer for novel self-healable wound dressing applications. *Macromolecular Materials and Engineering, 304*(3), 1800603.
3. Zielinski, J. M., & Duda, J. L. (1992). Predicting polymer/solvent diffusion coefficients using free-volume theory. *AIChE Journal, 38*(3), 405–415.

4. Duda, J. L., Vrentas, J. S., Ju, S. T., & Liu, H. T. (1982). Prediction of diffusion coefficients for polymer-solvent systems. *AIChE Journal, 28*(2), 279–285.
5. Vrentas, J. S., & Duda, J. L. (1977). Diffusion in polymer—solvent systems. I. Reexamination of the free-volume theory. *Journal of Polymer Science: Polymer Physics Edition, 15*(3), 403–416.
6. Vrentas, J. S., & Duda, J. L. (1977). Diffusion in polymer–solvent systems. II. A predictive theory for the dependence of diffusion coefficients on temperature, concentration, and molecular weight. *Journal of Polymer Science: Polymer Physics Edition, 15*(3), 417–439.
7. Flory, P. J. (1970). Fifteenth spiers memorial lecture. Thermodynamics of polymer solutions. *Discussions of the Faraday Society, 49*, 7–29.
8. Willis, J. D., Beardsley, T. M., & Matsen, M. W. (2020). Simple and accurate calibration of the Flory–Huggins interaction parameter. *Macromolecules, 53*(22), 9973–9982.
9. Liu, Y., Li, Y., Yang, G., Zheng, X., & Zhou, S. (2015). Multi-stimulus-responsive shape-memory polymer nanocomposite network cross-linked by cellulose nanocrystals. *ACS Applied Materials & Interfaces, 7*(7), 4118–4126.
10. Xiao, R., Guo, J., Safranski, D. L., & Nguyen, T. D. (2015). Solvent-driven temperature memory and multiple shape memory effects. *Soft Matter, 11*(20), 3977–3985.
11. Rana, M. M., Rajeev, A., Natale, G., & De la Hoz Siegler, H. (2021). Effects of synthesis-solvent polarity on the physicochemical and rheological properties of poly (N-isopropylacrylamide)(PNIPAm) hydrogels. *Journal of Materials Research and Technology, 13*, 769–786.
12. Metze, F. K., Sant, S., Meng, Z., Klok, H. A., & Kaur, K. (2023). Swelling-activated, soft mechanochemistry in polymer materials. *Langmuir, 39*(10), 3546–3557.
13. Bandyopadhyay, A., Dasgupta, P., & Basak, S. (2020). *Engineering of thermoplastic elastomer with graphene and other anisotropic nanofillers*. Springer.
14. Zhuo, S., Shu Hieng Tie, B., Keane, G., & Geever, L. M. (2023). Strategies for developing shape-shifting behaviours and potential applications of poly (N-vinyl Caprolactam) hydrogels. *Polymers, 15*(6), 1511.
15. Zhao, Y., Chun Wang, C., Min Huang, W., & Purnawali, H. (2011). Buckling of poly (methyl methacrylate) in stimulus-responsive shape recovery. *Appl. Phys. Lett.* 99, 131911.
16. Salvekar, A. V., Huang, W. M., Xiao, R., Wong, Y. S., Venkatraman, S. S., Tay, K. H., & Shen, Z. X. (2017). Water-responsive shape recovery induced buckling in biodegradable photo-cross-linked poly (ethylene glycol)(PEG) hydrogel. *Accounts of Chemical Research, 50*(2), 141–150.
17. Gu, X., & Mather, P. T. (2013). Water-triggered shape memory of multiblock thermoplastic polyurethanes (TPUs). *Rsc Advances, 3*(36), 15783–15791.
18. Vesely, D. (2001). Molecular sorption mechanism of solvent diffusion in polymers. *Polymer, 42*(9), 4417–4422.
19. Peppas, N. A., Gurny, R., Doelker, E., & Buri, P. (1980). Modelling of drug diffusion through swellable polymeric systems. *Journal of Membrane Science, 7*(3), 241–253.

20. Darvishmanesh, S., Buekenhoudt, A., Degrève, J., & Van der Bruggen, B. (2009). General model for prediction of solvent permeation through organic and inorganic solvent resistant nanofiltration membranes. *Journal of Membrane Science*, *334*(1–2), 43–49.

21. Felderhof, B. U., & Deutch, J. M. (1976). Concentration dependence of the rate of diffusion-controlled reactions. *The Journal of Chemical Physics*, *64*(11), 4551–4558.

22. Taylor, G. I. (1922). Diffusion by continuous movements. *Proceedings of the London Mathematical Society*, *2*(1), 196–212.

23. Krogh, A. (1919). The rate of diffusion of gases through animal tissues, with some remarks on the coefficient of invasion. *The Journal of Physiology*, *52*(6), 391.

Effects of Solvent on Thermomechanical Properties of Solvent- Responsive Shape Memory Polymer

5

In the realm of materials science and engineering, the extent to which a material absorbs a solvent, particularly in minute quantities, plays a pivotal role in influencing a property known as the glass transition temperature (T_g). This parameter holds significant importance as it delineates the material's capability to undergo a change in shape without necessitating the application of external heat—a phenomenon commonly referred to as athermal shape deployment [1–4].

The glass transition temperature serves as a critical threshold, delineating the transition between the material's rigid, glassy state and its more flexible, rubbery state. Materials exhibiting a T_g below ambient temperature are typically in a glassy state, characterized by a rigid molecular structure with limited mobility. Conversely, when the Tg exceeds ambient temperature, the material enters a rubbery state, wherein molecular motion becomes more pronounced, enabling shape change and deformation.

DOI: 10.1201/9781003593805-5

The concept of athermal shape deployment hinges on exploiting the unique properties of materials with T_g values strategically positioned within the operational temperature range. By judiciously selecting materials with suitable T_g values and incorporating solvent absorption mechanisms, engineers can design smart materials capable of undergoing reversible shape changes triggered solely by environmental cues, such as solvent exposure.

Understanding the intricate interplay between solvent absorption and the glass transition temperature is imperative for the development of advanced materials with tailored properties and functionalities. Such knowledge not only facilitates the design of innovative materials for diverse applications but also underscores the significance of solvent-polymer interactions in shaping the behavior and performance of engineered systems.

When a solvent seeps into a material, even just a little bit, it sets off a chain reaction of effects that greatly influence how the material behaves mechanically. One of the main ways this happens is by making the molecular chains in the material more mobile. This increased mobility happens because the solvent adds more possible ways for the molecules to arrange themselves, which reduces the time it takes for the material to transition from one state to another—known as the relaxation time—and causes the glass transition temperature to decrease.

Researchers have been working hard to refine models that explain this complex relationship between solvent and material behavior. One such model, the Adam-Gibbs model, was originally designed to describe how liquids behave when they're cooled below their freezing point. But scientists have adapted and improved it to better understand how solvents affect molecular movement and, ultimately, the glass transition temperature. This updated model helps us grasp how solvent molecules change a material's properties, which is invaluable for designing materials with specific characteristics [5].

Nguyen et al. recently brilliantly captured the comprehensive model that has been incorporated into finite element analysis, allowing the development of precisely customized computational models to explore the isothermal recovery behavior of specimens exposed to both air and water environments [5]. These models were created to account for the complex diffusion process, resulting in an accurate simulation of the actual healing process. Furthermore, empirical studies strongly confirm the constitutive model's prediction accuracy. It accurately predicts the saturated material's considerable softening of the stress response and elucidates the time-dependent, solvent-driven shape recovery process. This achievement demonstrates the created model's robustness in understanding the solvent-driven shape memory effect.

Delving into the exploration of how solvents impact the thermomechanical properties of solvent-responsive SMPs within biomedical applications prompts an intriguing question. Why do we embark on this journey? To grasp the answer, it's crucial to first understand the significant role that shape memory polymers (SMPs) play in the biomedical arena [6].

SMP devices are meticulously crafted to serve precise functions within biomedical applications. They are engineered to exhibit shape memory behavior, meaning they can be temporarily deformed into intricate shapes and then recover their original shape when triggered by specific stimuli. This ability is invaluable in various biomedical scenarios, where precise control over shape change and recovery trajectories is essential [6–8].

SMP devices are frequently designed in biomedical applications to acquire complicated temporary shapes and recovery trajectories. This research project has the potential to contribute significantly to the design process by providing predictive insights into the influence of shape memory programming processes and deployment conditions, such as temperature and solvent properties, on shape recovery dynamics [9–11]. It is worth mentioning that the polymer under consideration in this work has a proclivity for absorbing only modest amounts of solvent, with the resulting solvent-driven recovery taking hours. In the future, the researchers hope to investigate polymer systems with a high proclivity for solvent absorption and quick diffusion kinetics. To achieve this goal, a fully coupled thermodynamic theory capable of capturing the complicated interplay between mechanical and diffusion processes will need to be developed [9–11].

Nguyen et al. beautifully capture these various phenomena namely the variation in the isothermal stress response and in the case of isothermal recovery.

Figure 5.1 depicts a comparison of experimental observations and simulations of stress–strain behavior (of a meth(acrylate) copolymer network) in isothermal, uniaxial tension tests performed at ambient temperature. The research differentiates between dry and moist specimens. The dry specimen, in particular, exhibited a standard hard glassy response with a clear yield point, subsequent softening after yielding, and a viscoplastic flow phase. In contrast, as expected, the saturated specimen exhibited more pliable rubbery behavior with no evident yield point [3]. This opposite behavior can be explained by the penetration of solvent molecules in the polymer matrix. As a result, the transition temperature of the glass drops below the room temperature. This softens the saturated specimen's stress–strain response significantly. The simulation results are very similar to the experimental data. However, it is important to note that the model slightly underestimates the saturated specimen stress response. One possible explanation for this difference could be due to hydration loss during the experimental process [5].

Similarly, in Figure 5.2, the illustration provides a visual representation of the investigation conducted on the shape memory cycle of dry uniaxial tension specimens, encompassing both the programming and isothermal

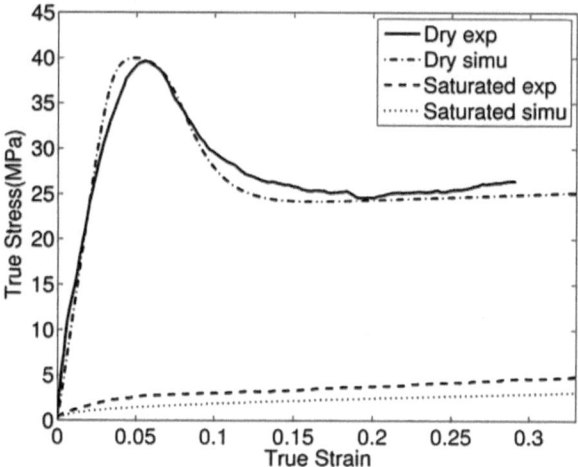

FIGURE 5.1   The stress–strain response for dry and saturated specimens at room temperature. Reproduced with permission from [5], copyright reserved Royal Society of Chemistry 2013.

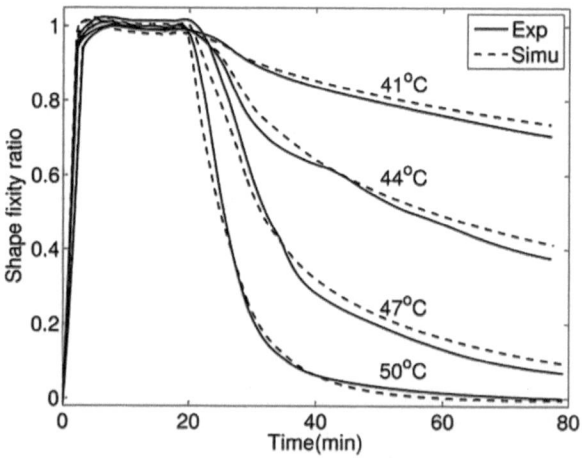

FIGURE 5.2   The experimental and simulation results for shape memory programming and isothermal, unconstrained recovery of tension specimens in air. Reproduced with permission from [5], copyright reserved Royal Society of Chemistry 2013.

recovery phases. The assessment of shape recovery was quantitatively undertaken by measuring the reduction in the shape fixity ratio [5].

The data analysis revealed a clear and consistent trend: as the recovery temperature rose, so did the recovery time. For instance, at 41°C, less than 30% of the deformation was regained after an hour. However, at 50°C, complete recovery was achieved in just 15 minutes. This observation underscores the direct relationship between recovery temperature and the efficiency of shape recovery.

In the specific case of the dry methacrylate network material, programmed specimens exhibited impressive resistance to recovery even after prolonged storage at room temperature. This resilience suggests the material's stability and reliability in maintaining its programmed shape over time. However, when these same programmed specimens were submerged in water for extended periods, a significant loss of shape fixation was observed. This highlights the material's susceptibility to environmental factors, such as moisture, which can compromise its shape memory properties [3–5].

Similarly, as we turn our attention to Figure 5.3, it presents a graphical depiction of the shape fixity ratio during the isothermal recovery process of specimens that had been immersed in water at two specific temperatures: 25°C and 30°C. What merits particular attention in this context is the

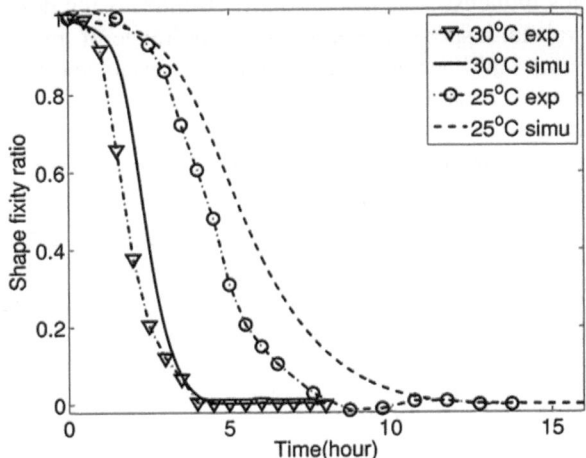

FIGURE 5.3 The experimental and simulation results for isothermal, unconstrained recovery of tension specimens in water. Reproduced with permission from [5], copyright reserved Royal Society of Chemistry 2013.

noteworthy observation that these specimens, when subjected to these precise temperature conditions, demonstrated the remarkable capability to restore their original dimensions completely. To provide precise temporal context, it is worth noting that this process of recovery was accomplished within a time frame of 8 hours at 25°C and a mere 4 hours at 30°C [3,5].

Figure 5.4 provides an in-depth visual representation of another critical aspect of our investigation: the macroscopic shape recovery of methacrylate-based SMP. As discussed earlier, this macroscopic recovery is closely tied to two fundamental phenomena: the noticeable softening of the stress response seen in the saturated material and the time-dependent shape recovery driven by solvent effects [5–8].

This correlation is rooted in the intricate interplay between solvent diffusion and kinetics, a topic thoroughly explored in our study. As more solvent permeates the polymer matrix, it brings about significant changes in the material's thermomechanical properties [9–11]. This transformation essentially sets the stage for stress softening, a phenomenon that greatly facilitates the subsequent shape recovery of the polymer. In essence, the entry of solvent into the polymer matrix plays a pivotal role in reshaping the material's thermomechanical landscape, acting as a precursor to its ability to revert to its original shape [12–14].

Understanding this complex process is not only academically significant but also holds immense practical relevance. It informs the design and engineering of solvent-responsive SMPs for a wide range of applications. This underscores the multifaceted nature of these materials and their promising potential in various technological and biomedical contexts.

Expanding on this theme the relationship between diffusion rate, permeation, and temperature during sorption and desorption processes demonstrates

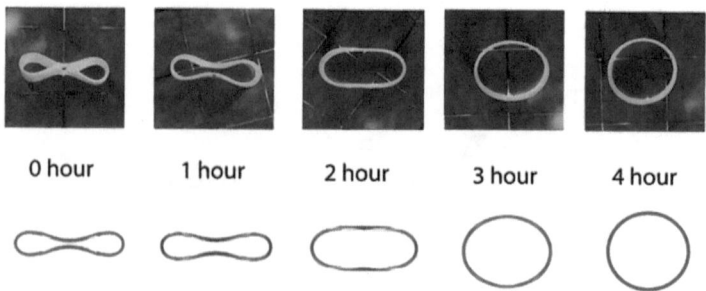

| 0 hour | 1 hour | 2 hour | 3 hour | 4 hour |

FIGURE 5.4   The instantaneous configuration of tube specimens observed in both experimental and simulated conditions within a water bath maintained at a temperature of 30°C. Reproduced with permission from [5], copyright reserved Royal Society of Chemistry 2013.

a clear dependency, as discussed in reference [15]. Evaluating the activation energy of diffusion involves analyzing its temperature dependency using the Arrhenius law, expressed as:

$$D = D_0 \exp\left[-\frac{E_a}{R\theta}\right] \tag{5.1}$$

Here, (E_a) represents the activation energy, (θ) is the absolute temperature, and (R) is the universal gas constant (equal to 8.314 J/mol·K).

Figure 5.5 presents a plot of $(\ln(D))$ versus (θ) for three solvents studied. This graph reveals an almost linear relationship for Estane (thermoplastic polyurethane)-solvent samples across the temperature range. By conducting regression analysis on these plots, we can calculate the apparent activation energies (E_a) of diffusion for acetone, ethanol, and water as 32, 58.3, and 56.5 kJ/mol, respectively.

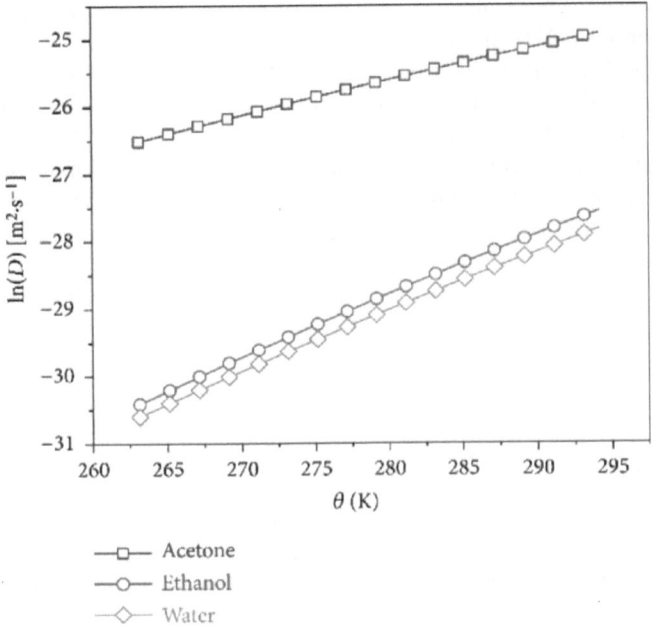

FIGURE 5.5 The temperature dependency of diffusion coefficients of three different solvents (acetone, ethanol, and water) inside Estane to demonstrate the dependence of ln(D) versus for the sorption process. The data are obtained from experimental weight gain measurements. Reproduced with permission from [16], copyright reserved Hindawi 2018.

These findings are consistent with activation energies observed for similar small molecules in polyurethanes, as reported in the related literature [16]. The analysis of activation energy provides valuable insights into the temperature sensitivity of diffusion processes, contributing to our understanding of how molecular mobility and interactions within polymers are influenced by temperature variations. This data aids in predicting and optimizing sorption and desorption behaviors in polymer-solvent systems under different environmental conditions.

In addition to diffusivity, the cohesive energy density (CED) and Hildebrand's solubility parameter play crucial roles in understanding and predicting permeability of sorbents in polymer samples, as discussed by Cavicchi and coworkers [17]. Hildebrand's solubility parameter (δ) is a numerical measure that indicates the strength of molecular interactions between solvents and polymers. Materials with similar solubility parameters tend to dissolve in each other more readily.

On the other hand, CED can be described as the total energy required to completely separate a unit volume of material from its neighbors to an infinite distance. This value can be determined, for example, through molecular dynamics (MD) simulations by calculating the energy increase per mole of material when all intermolecular forces cease [20]. The derivation of CED typically relies on three primary solubility parameters introduced by Hildebrand and Scott [16].

Furthermore, Hansen's approach extends beyond simply addressing hydrogen bonding (H-bonds) to integrate a broader range of interactions. This comprehensive understanding of CED and solubility parameters allows for a more nuanced assessment of how different types of molecular interactions influence the permeability and compatibility of solvents with polymers [16]. These parameters serve as valuable tools for predicting and evaluating the interactions between polymers and solvents, aiding in the design and optimization of polymer compositions for various applications. The integration of CED and solubility parameters provides critical insights into the behavior of polymer-solvent systems, facilitating informed decisions in materials science and engineering.

The solubility characteristics of polyurethane are distinctly weak in water but notably better in acetone or ethanol, suggesting a stronger affinity of polyurethane (Estane) toward ethanol or acetone over water. Additionally, the permeability and solubility parameters exhibit a similar magnitude or order of magnitude, reinforcing the preferential interaction of polyurethane with ethanol or acetone.

Furthermore, the thermodynamic parameters governing diffusion can be assessed using Van't Hoff's relation [18]:

$$\log K_s = \left(\frac{\Delta S}{2.303R} \right) - \left(\frac{\Delta H}{2.303R\theta} \right) \tag{5.2}$$

Here, ΔH and ΔS represent the changes in enthalpy and entropy, respectively, and K_s is the equilibrium sorption constant. This constant can be estimated using the following equation:

$$K_s = \frac{n_s^{sp}}{m_p} \tag{5.3}$$

where (n_s^{sp}) denotes the number of moles of the sorbed solvent at equilibrium and m is the mass of the sorbent. The values of ΔH and ΔS can be obtained from the slope and intercept of the plot of ln K versus $1/\theta$.

In the context of sorption, the values of ΔH are positive for all sorbents and fall within the range of 0.0267–0.06 kJ/mol. These positive ΔH values indicate endothermic sorption processes dominated by the Fickian mode, likely due to the creation of new pores within the sample during sorption.

This comprehensive analysis of thermodynamic parameters not only elucidates the energy requirements and driving forces governing sorption processes but also offers valuable insights into the behavior and characteristics of polymer-solvent interactions. Understanding these interactions is pivotal for optimizing material design and comprehending transport phenomena within polymeric systems.

These insights directly correlate with the way solvent-responsive SMPs interact with and absorb solvents, ultimately triggering their responsive behavior. The ability of these polymers to selectively absorb specific solvents, such as ethanol or acetone over water, aligns with their affinity and permeability characteristics toward certain chemical environments.

By leveraging knowledge of thermodynamic parameters, such as activation energies, CED, Hildebrand's solubility parameter, and changes in enthalpy (ΔH) and entropy (ΔS) during sorption, engineers and researchers can tailor solvent-responsive SMPs to exhibit precise and controlled responses to environmental stimuli. This includes designing polymers that contract, expand, or undergo shape transformations based on solvent interactions, enabling applications in fields ranging from biomedical devices to smart textiles and responsive coatings.

In essence, the deep understanding of polymer-solvent interactions gleaned from these analyses is instrumental in harnessing the full potential of solvent-responsive SMPs [19–21]. This knowledge not only informs material design strategies but also opens new avenues for innovation in responsive and adaptive polymer technologies.

REFERENCES

1. Kroon-Batenburg, L. M. J., & Kroon, J. (1990). Solvent effect on the conformation of the hydroxymethyl group established by molecular dynamics simulations of methyl-β-D-glucoside in water. *Biopolymers: Original Research on Biomolecules, 29*(8–9), 1243–1248.
2. Thomas, K. R., Chenneviere, A., Reiter, G., & Steiner, U. (2011). Nonequilibrium behavior of thin polymer films. *Physical Review E, 83*(2), 021804.
3. Simha, R., & Boyer, R. F. (1962). On a general relation involving the glass temperature and coefficients of expansion of polymers. *The Journal of Chemical Physics, 37*(5), 1003–1007.
4. Bain, D. F., Munday, D. L., & Smith, A. (1999). Solvent influence on spray-dried biodegradable microspheres. *Journal of Microencapsulation, 16*(4), 453–474.
5. Xiao, R., & Nguyen, T. D. (2013). Modeling the solvent-induced shape-memory behavior of glassy polymers. *Soft Matter, 9*(39), 9455–9464.
6. Nadgorny, M., & Ameli, A. (2018). Functional polymers and nanocomposites for 3D printing of smart structures and devices. *ACS Applied Materials & Interfaces, 10*(21), 17489–17507.
7. Basak, S., & Bandyopadhyay, A. (2022). Styrene-butadiene-styrene-based shape memory polymers: Evolution and the current state of art. *Polymers for Advanced Technologies, 33*(7), 2091–2112.
8. Basak, S. (2021). Redesigning the modern applied medical sciences and engineering with shape memory polymers. *Advanced Composites and Hybrid Materials, 4*, 223–234.
9. Yakacki, C. M., & Gall, K. (2010). Shape-memory polymers for biomedical applications. Shape-memory polymers, *Advances in Polymer Science, 226*(1), 147–175.
10. Biswas, A., Singh, A. P., Rana, D., Aswal, V. K., & Maiti, P. (2018). Biodegradable toughened nanohybrid shape memory polymer for smart biomedical applications. *Nanoscale, 10*(21), 9917–9934.
11. Yahia, L. (2015). Introduction to shape-memory polymers for biomedical applications. L'Hocine Yahia (Ed.), In *Shape memory polymers for biomedical applications* (pp. 3–8). Woodhead Publishing.
12. Ecker, M., Danda, V., Shoffstall, A. J., Mahmood, S. F., Joshi-Imre, A., Frewin, C. L., … & Voit, W. E. (2017). Sterilization of thiol-ene/acrylate based shape memory polymers for biomedical applications. *Macromolecular Materials and Engineering, 302*(2), 1600331.
13. Pisani, S., Genta, I., Modena, T., Dorati, R., Benazzo, M., & Conti, B. (2022). Shape-memory polymers hallmarks and their biomedical applications in the form of nanofibers. *International Journal of Molecular Sciences, 23*(3), 1290.
14. Huang, W. M., Yang, B., Zhao, Y., & Ding, Z. (2010). Thermo-moisture responsive polyurethane shape-memory polymer and composites: A review. *Journal of Materials Chemistry, 20*(17), 3367–3381.
15. Burke, J. (1984). Solubility parameters: Theory and application. Available at https://cool.culturalheritage.org/coolaic/sg/bpg/annual/v03/bp03-04.html

16. Ghobadi, E., Marquardt, A., Zirdehi, E. M., Neuking, K., Varnik, F., Eggeler, G., & Steeb, H. (2018). The influence of water and solvent uptake on functional properties of shape-memory polymers. *International Journal of Polymer Science*, *2018*(1), 7819353.

17. Basak, S., & Cavicchi, K. A. (2023). Structure–property relationships of shape memory, semicrystalline polymers fabricated by in situ polymerization and crosslinking of octadecyl acrylate/polybutadiene blends. *Macromolecular Rapid Communications*, *44*(1), 2200404.

18. Ghobadi, E., Heuchel, M., Kratz, K., & Lendlein, A. (2012). Simulation of volumetric swelling of degradable poly [(rac-lactide)-co-glycolide] based polyesterurethanes containing different urethane-linkers. *Journal of Applied Biomaterials & Functional Materials*, *10*(3), 293–301.

19. Lu, H. (2013). State diagram of phase transition temperatures and solvent-induced recovery behavior of shape-memory polymer. *Journal of Applied Polymer Science*, *127*(4), 2896–2904.

20. Aitken, H. M., Jiang, Z., Hampton, I., O'Mara, M. L., & Connal, L. A. (2022). Polymer–solvent interactions as a tool to engineer material properties. *Molecular Systems Design & Engineering*, *7*(7), 746–754.

21. Guo, Q., Zhang, Y., Ruan, H., Sun, H., Wang, T., Wang, Q., & Wang, C. (2024). Solvent content controlling strategy for cocrystallizable polyesters enables a stress-free two-way shape memory effect with wider service temperatures. *Macromolecular Rapid Communications*, *45*(3), 2300534.

Emerging Applications of Solvent-Responsive Shape Memory Polymers in Biomedical Applications

6

6.1 APPLICATION IN POLYMER STENTS

Since its inception, there has been a considerable amount of attention directed toward the advancement of biomedical devices and implants that exhibit sensitivity to solvents, all with the primary objective of eliminating the need for heat-based activation. Typically, metallic stents are limited in their ability to endure elastic deformation, typically up to 10%, beyond which point they lose their elasticity, and this is where polymers appear to be an apt alternative to the problem [1–3].

DOI: 10.1201/9781003593805-6

In the realm of vascular interventions, metallic stents have long served as effective tools for mitigating acute occlusion and reducing late restenosis following coronary angioplasty. However, despite their undeniable merits, a constellation of concerns continues to shadow their usage. In this context, attention is directed toward an intriguing alternative: poly-l-lactic acid (PLLA) stents. Diverging from their metallic counterparts, PLLA stents possess distinctive attributes, most notably their biodegradable nature and the capability to deliver therapeutic agents locally [4]. The primary objective of this study was to conduct a thorough evaluation of PLLA stents, with a principal focus on their feasibility, safety, and efficacy within clinical applications. This endeavor represents a pivotal advancement in the quest for innovative solutions in vascular interventions. The unique properties of PLLA stents (Figure 6.1), particularly their biodegradability and drug delivery potential, open up a promising avenue for addressing enduring challenges and reservations associated with metallic stents.

Wang et al. first introduced the idea of shape memory in polymers stents in 2006, a concept that would later prove to be a game-changer in the world of responsive polymer. In the last ten years, biodegradable stents have gained a lot of attention. This is because stents serve a temporary purpose when implanted in the human body. In response to this observation, researchers have explored the development of fully polymer stents. One of the most prominent examples of this is the Igaki-Tamai stent (Figure 6.1). This stent is made from poly (i.e., l-lactide or PLLA). It has been shown to be safe and effective in human applications. One notable limitation of the stent is that it needs to be heated to 70°C to self-expand. This process may cause cellular trauma during deployment [4]. The imperative for such heating stems from the fact that mere balloon expansion of the stent does not guarantee its secure anchoring [5–7]. Unlike metal stents, which undergo plastic deformation

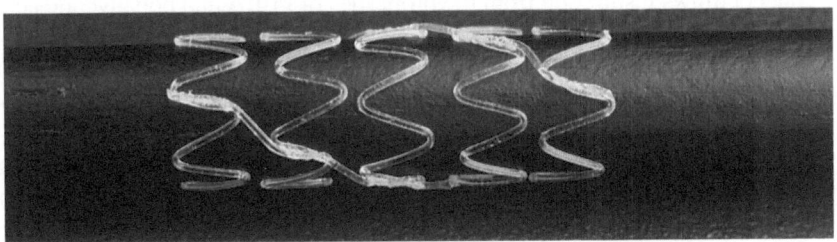

FIGURE 6.1   The Igaki-Tamai stent is a premounted, balloon-expandable PLLA stent that also has the ability of self-expansion. Reproduced with permission from [4], copyright reserved American Heart Organisation 2000.

during expansion, most polymers with suitable mechanical properties tend to recoil immediately after balloon expansion. This property is undesirable for stent deployment in vascular settings and can even pose life-threatening risks in the case of coronary stents. Consequently, fully polymeric stents must possess a degree of self-expandability to exert a gentle outward force against the vessel wall, anchoring themselves securely. In this context, self-expandability denotes the intrinsic ability to expand without the requirement of an external force [7].

Two predominant methodologies have been pursued to achieve self-expandability in fully polymeric stents: the sheath method and the incorporation of elastic memory. In the sheath method, the initially expanded stent is enclosed within a sheath, which is subsequently removed using a specialized catheter upon reaching the intended deployment site. Alternatively, some designs involve a sheath consisting of a thin chitosan coating, anticipated to degrade within the body upon contact with moisture, thereby liberating the stent. However, this approach necessitates a meticulous balance between the rate of sheath disintegration and the stent's deployment timeline to avoid premature or delayed expansion [5].

The most desirable approach would involve anchoring stents through a self-expansion mechanism at the body's natural temperature. While this concept is theoretically feasible through the use of crosslinked polymers, it's important to recognize that the development of a new crosslinked biodegradable polymer would require an extensive series of safety studies. These studies are critical for ensuring the safety and effectiveness of the polymer, but they also inevitably lead to an elongated development timeline [5–7].

To overcome this formidable challenge, Dr. Wang and his dedicated research group have strategically leveraged well-established biodegradable polymers. Their innovative solution involves the creation of a novel multilayered stent that incorporates a concept known as partial elastic memory. This concept draws inspiration from the properties of PLLA and polyglycolic acid (PLGA) polymers, both widely recognized in the field of biomedical materials. This groundbreaking innovation allows for a relatively swift and efficient self-expansion mechanism to occur within the human body, all at physiological temperatures. The patented bi-layered prototype stent, meticulously conceived within our laboratory under Dr. Wang's guidance, offers a promising resolution to the intricate challenge of achieving self-expandability without the need for external heating [5]. Illustrated in Figure 6.2, this remarkable development signifies a significant step forward in the realm of stent technology. It not only holds the potential to enhance the safety and efficacy of stent deployment but also offers the prospect of expediting the translation of this cutting-edge technology into practical clinical applications. Dr. Wang's

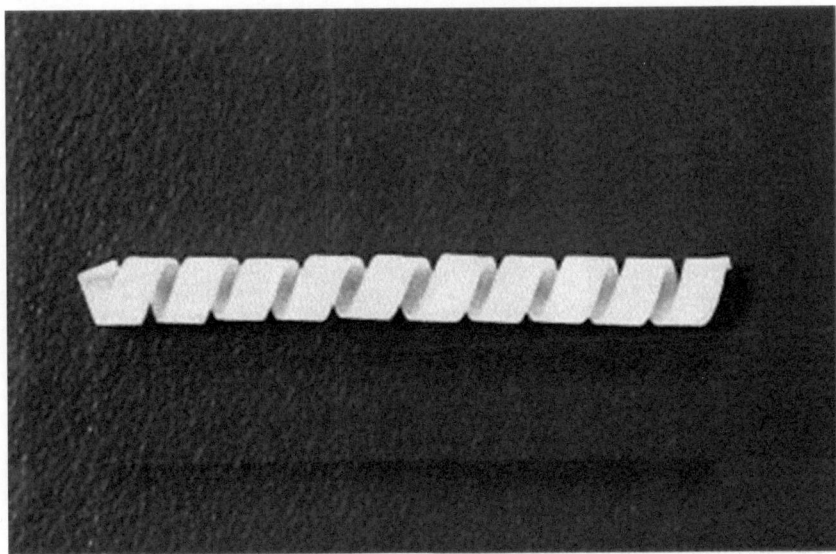

FIGURE 6.2   Photograph of helicoidal stent prototype. Reproduced with permission from [5], copyright reserved Elsevier 2006.

pioneering work in this area underscores the importance of innovation and creative problem-solving in advancing medical science.

Although there had been a significant effort to synthesize polymeric stents, the use of thermoresponsive polymers was a major concern, in terms of its practical applicability. Among the early breakthroughs in this field, Dr. Chen and his dedicated research team introduced a pioneering innovation. They formulated a composite material consisting of an epoxy matrix blended with glycerol, poly(ethylene oxide), and chitosan, envisioning its application as a self-expanding stent [8]. However, Chen et al. managed to push the boundaries by demonstrating that their developed polymer blend could undergo deformation of nearly 30% strain and still revert to its original shape when exposed to a specific stimulus, such as water. This remarkable achievement was confirmed through a comprehensive animal study.

It is pertinent to emphasize that the epoxy compound employed in our research features flexible ether bonds $(-O-)$ that function as pliable junctions within the cross-linking bridges. Notably, prior research conducted by Lohre et al. has effectively established that the cytotoxicity profile of epoxy compounds is substantially more favorable than that of glutaraldehyde [9], thus rendering epoxy compounds a viable and acceptable fixative agent in

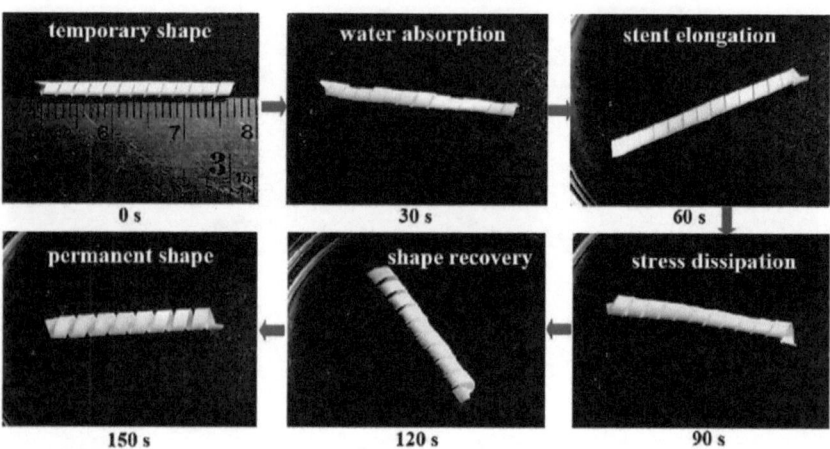

FIGURE 6.3   Images capturing the progression of the polymeric (Chitosan/glycerol/Polyethylene oxide) stent's self-expansion over time, while it is submerged in a phosphate-buffered saline solution and activated through the process of hydration. Reproduced with permission from [8], copyright reserved American Chemical Society 2007.

the production of implantable devices, contingent upon maintaining residual levels below cytotoxic thresholds.

The chemically crosslinked polymers resulting from these processes yield insoluble materials that exhibit significant swelling when exposed to an aqueous environment. As graphically depicted in Figure 6.3, the stent, in its desiccated (crimped) state, progressively reverts to its permanent shape over a period of time upon hydration, ultimately reaching an equilibrium state. Upon achieving this permanent configuration (typically within a mere 150 seconds), the mobility and flow of polymer chains cease, primarily due to the presence of crosslinkage points situated within these polymer chains. These crosslinkage points function as anchoring entities or "permanent entanglements," effectively preventing the chains from undergoing relative slippage [9].

Therefore, the administration of an external stimulus—specifically, hydration—can cause the stent to change from its temporary shape (when it is dehydrated and crimped) to its permanent condition (upon full expansion). It is also important to note that this transformation process is entirely reversible, as illustrated visually in Figure 6.4. Due to this unique property, the new polymeric stent can be implanted into an artery using minimally invasive surgical techniques in a crimped (temporary) structure and then extended to take on a permanent configuration as needed.

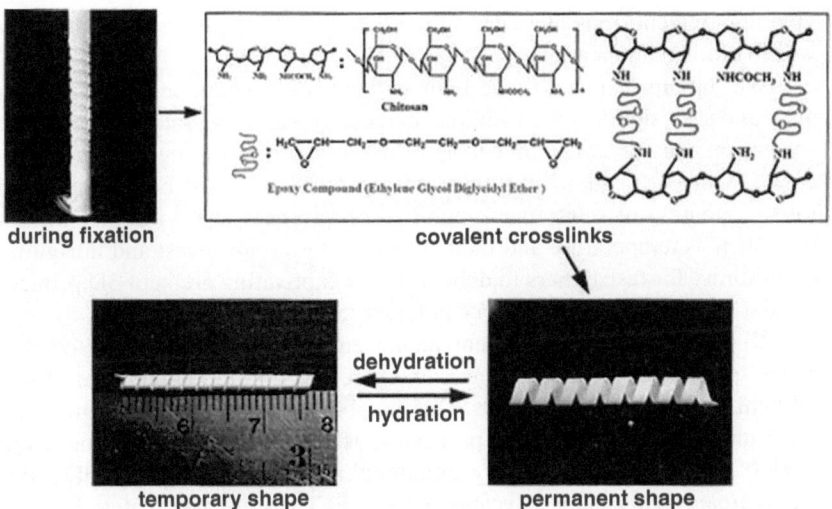

during fixation   covalent crosslinks

temporary shape   permanent shape

FIGURE 6.4   Cross-linking structures and photographs of the permanent and temporary shapes of the polymeric (Chitosan/glycerol/polyethylene oxide) stent. The shape-switching process is reversible and controlled by hydration or dehydration of the crosslinked stent. Reproduced with permission from [8], copyright reserved American Chemical Society 2007.

Significantly, it is imperative to note that the self-expansion process of the developed stent, as it transitions from its crimped state to its permanent state, has been meticulously examined and found to occur within a remarkably brief timeframe, specifically 150 ± 10 seconds at a temperature of 37°C. This rapid transition represents a substantial advancement when juxtaposed with the self-expansion periods exhibited by polymeric stents fabricated from PLLA (approximately 20 minutes at 37°C for the Igaki–Tamai stent) [4] or PLLA/PLGA (approximately 8 minutes at 37°C for the stent developed by Venkatraman et al.) [5].

The pronounced divergence in these self-expansion durations can be attributed to a fundamental dissimilarity in the triggering mechanisms. Notably, our developed stent responds to hydration, effectively bypassing the need for external thermal induction. Furthermore, it is worth emphasizing that the choice of raw materials employed in the fabrication of our stent— chitosan and polyethylene oxide—confers upon it a relatively high hydrophilicity. This inherent property renders the stent exceptionally responsive to hydration, contributing significantly to its expeditious self-expandability. The expeditious nature of this self-expansion process carries profound advantages, particularly in terms of mitigating the risk of stent migration during in vivo deployment, thus augmenting the safety and effectiveness of the stent within clinical applications.

We anticipate that this domain will not only continue to expand but also undergo significant evolution, extending its reach into the realm of solvent-responsive stents, amenable to manufacturing through additive processes. Currently, additive manufacturing techniques are being harnessed for the creation of stents that exhibit responsiveness to environmental factors, such as temperature and light. This trend presents a vast and intriguing opportunity for researchers to delve into the captivating arena of 3D printed, solvent-responsive shape memory polymer (SMP) stents.

To delve deeper into recent advancements in crafting bioresorbable stents, innovative techniques have emerged, pushing the boundaries of traditional manufacturing methods. One notable approach involves combining 3D printing with spray-coating processes, as demonstrated by the pioneering work of Park et al. [10]. In their groundbreaking research, they used 3D printing to create stents using polycaprolactone (PCL) as the base material.

What makes their work stand out is the subsequent application of a specialized coating made from a blend of poly(lactic-co-glycolic acid) (PLGA) and poly(ethylene glycol) (PEG). This strategic blend serves a dual purpose: it not only strengthens the structure of the stent but also enables the controlled release of sirolimus, a potent drug used to prevent restenosis—undesirable narrowing of blood vessels after stent implantation.

By combining the versatility of 3D printing with the precision of spray-coating techniques, Park et al. have brought about a significant change in stent manufacturing. This innovative approach not only provides better control over stent composition and drug delivery but also opens up possibilities for personalized treatment strategies, catering to the unique needs of individual patients.

What we understand that their pioneering research represents a major step forward in the field of bioresorbable stents, offering new possibilities for personalized, effective, and minimally invasive cardiovascular interventions. By seamlessly integrating cutting-edge technologies with biomaterials, Park et al. have transformed the landscape of stent design and manufacturing, offering renewed hope for patients worldwide.

In certain instances, researchers have turned to injection molding techniques to produce bioresorbable stents composed of poly(l-lactide-co-glycolide-co-trimethylene carbonate). These stents exhibit a remarkable attribute of rapid self-expansion within a matter of seconds, albeit at a temperature slightly above the physiological range, typically at 41°C [11]. This expedited self-expansion holds considerable promise for enhancing the efficiency of stent deployment within the body. Moreover, some research groups have ventured into uncharted territory by incorporating pressure sensors into their stent designs. This innovative approach enables real-time monitoring of stent absorption over time, affording a deeper understanding of the dynamics of resorption and the consequential alterations in stent properties within the living organism.

Taking a different trajectory, Hollister et al. have embarked on the design and production of airway stents based on PCL through the selective laser sintering method. These stents have demonstrated significant potential in ameliorating pulmonary and extrapulmonary conditions associated with tracheobronchomalacia, especially in pediatric patients [12]. Of particular significance is the observation of continued tissue growth within the airways over an extended duration, a testament to the deliberate design of these stents with controlled degradation in mind [12].

Collectively, these diverse and innovative approaches underscore the dynamic and ever-evolving landscape of bioresorbable stent development. Each technique brings with it unique advantages and insights, pushing the boundaries of what is achievable in this field and holding the promise of improved patient care and outcomes. Readers are recommended to peruse a beautifully crafted perspective by Dr. Becker, which provides a captivating and enlightening view of the realm of additive manufacturing and how it caters to the stent industry [13].

6.2 APPLICATION IN TISSUE SCAFFOLDS

Tissue scaffolds play a pivotal role in the field of tissue engineering, serving as fundamental devices designed to address the repair and regeneration of lost or damaged tissues. These scaffolds are subjected to a set of overarching requirements, which are essential for their effectiveness in the context of tissue engineering [14]. Polymer tissue scaffolds have been gaining substantial attention in the field of tissue engineering for several compelling reasons. One of the foremost factors contributing to this heightened interest is the versatility they offer in material selection. Polymers provide a wide range of options with varying properties, enabling researchers to tailor scaffolds to the specific requirements of different tissues and applications. Another pivotal attribute is the biodegradability of many polymers used in tissue scaffolds. These polymers can undergo natural degradation over time into non-toxic byproducts. This aligns seamlessly with the need for scaffolds to degrade gradually as new tissue develops, ensuring structural support during tissue regeneration and gradual dissipation as native tissue matures [15]. Biocompatibility is a hallmark characteristic of polymer-based scaffolds.

They exhibit a high degree of compatibility with the body, minimizing the risk of adverse reactions or inflammation upon implantation. This inherent biocompatibility creates a conducive environment for cellular attachment, proliferation, and tissue growth.

The utilization of SMPs in the realm of tissue scaffolds represents a significant advancement over conventional polymeric scaffolds. Two pivotal advantages underscore the transformative potential of SMPs in tissue engineering [16].

Firstly, SMP scaffolds possess the remarkable capability to dynamically change their shape over time. This dynamic attribute enables them to emulate the intricate and evolving behaviors observed within in vivo environments, mirroring the dynamic nature of tissues during the healing process [17]. As tissues undergo natural changes and adaptations, SMP scaffolds flex and adapt in response, ensuring they remain in perfect sync with the tissue's evolving needs. This dynamic shape adaptation introduces a new dimension of biomimicry, enhancing the scaffold's ability to facilitate natural and effective tissue regeneration [17].

Secondly, SMP scaffolds can be meticulously programmed into compact shapes, revolutionizing the landscape of minimally invasive surgical procedures. These pre-programmed scaffolds can be introduced into the body using minimally invasive techniques, such as laparoscopy or arthroscopy. This minimally invasive approach not only minimizes surgical trauma but also accelerates post-operative recovery, reducing pain and shortening hospital stays. Furthermore, these SMP scaffolds exhibit a remarkable ability to conform seamlessly to irregular tissue boundaries or defects. Their capacity to adjust their shape to precisely match the unique contours of the tissue defect enhances the integration of the scaffold with the surrounding tissue. This not only optimizes the support provided but also promotes efficient tissue regeneration, ultimately leading to enhanced patient outcomes and a higher quality of life. In essence, the integration of SMPs into tissue scaffolds heralds a new era in tissue engineering, one where dynamic adaptability and minimally invasive approaches converge to prioritize patient well-being and functional restoration [18].

We shall now look at the major contribution of solvent-responsive SMPs in the niche of tissue scaffolds. In the dynamic field of biomaterials and tissue engineering, the exploration of SMPs has been a journey marked by significant milestones and innovative breakthroughs. One such pivotal moment in this journey can be traced back to 2014 when the Lourdin research group introduced a revolutionary SMP created through the extrusion cooking of potato starch with glycerol. This pioneering material exhibited a remarkable shape recovery rate, exceeding 90%. What truly set it apart was its rapidity, with approximately 80% of the shape recovery occurring in less than

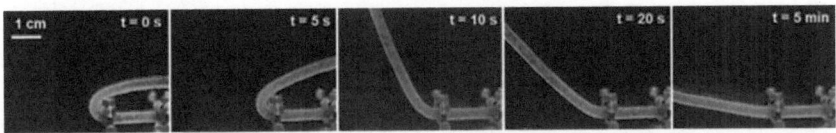

FIGURE 6.5 Time-course of the extruded starch shape recovery followed by images acquisition. Self-deployment of a straight shape memory extruded starch samples immersed in water at 37 C. Reproduced with permission from [19], copyright reserved Elsevier 2014.

20 seconds when immersed in water at a physiological temperature of 37°C (Figure 6.5) [19]. This remarkable SMP's true potential came to light when it was put to the test in a rat model. Here, it demonstrated not only its impressive shape memory properties but also its compatibility with living tissue. The scaffold showcased remarkable tissue integration capabilities, seamlessly fusing with the surrounding biological environment. Equally notable was the minimal inflammatory response elicited by this SMP, confirming its biocompatibility. This achievement opened up exciting avenues in the fields of tissue regeneration and drug delivery as it laid the foundation for scaffolds capable of mimicking the dynamic behaviors of living tissues.

Another remarkable innovation in the field of SMPs involved the creation of genipin crosslinked chitosan scaffolds. These sophisticated scaffolds possessed a unique capability to revert to their original shape even when immersed in water-ethanol mixtures. The presence of high ethanol content within the mixture induced dehydration of the matrix, allowing the amorphous vitreous network, predominantly composed of chitosan, to retain its temporary shape.

However, the introduction of water disrupted the hydrogen bonds responsible for large-scale segmental motion, thereby facilitating the shape recovery process. Remarkably, these scaffolds demonstrated outstanding shape fixity and shape recovery ratios of 99.2% and 98.5%, respectively. These exceptional properties, combined with their potential for minimally invasive implantation, rendered them highly suitable for a wide range of biomedical applications, spanning from tissue regeneration to drug delivery (as depicted in Figure 6.6).

In more recent years, the exploration of novel polymer systems, exemplified by poly(butanetetrol fumarate), has taken center stage in the development of intelligent SMPs [21]. These advanced materials have unlocked new dimensions in the fabrication of scaffolds with tailored properties, revolutionizing the field of biomaterials. Poly(butanetetrol fumarate) stands out for its exceptional solvent-induced shape memory properties, boasting shape fixity and shape recovery rates that surpass 95% (Figure 6.7). Beyond its shape

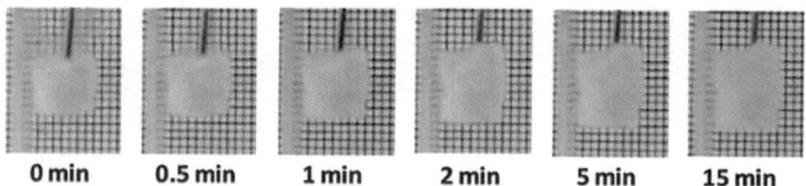

| 0 min | 0.5 min | 1 min | 2 min | 5 min | 15 min |

FIGURE 6.6   Series of photographs demonstrating the shape recovery process for genipin crosslinked chitosan scaffolds; the refereed times indicate the immersion time in water upon deformation at maximum strain = 30% and dehydration. Reproduced with permission from [20], copyright reserved Royal Society of Chemistry 2014.

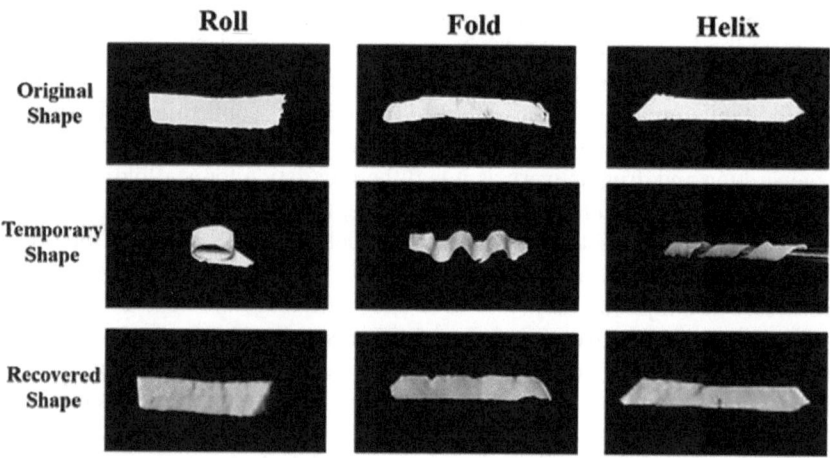

FIGURE 6.7   Water-responsive shape memory effect of PBF scaffolds from various temporary shapes. Reproduced with permission from [21], copyright reserved Royal Society of Chemistry 2019.

memory attributes, this polymer has demonstrated outstanding biodegradability, which not only promotes better cell attachment but also enhances cell viability and alkaline phosphatase activity (APA) of osteoblasts [21].

The polymer's biocompatibility was vividly demonstrated as cell adhesion increased significantly within just two to four hours, with an impressive 93.3 ± 16.3% cell adhesion ability. Furthermore, cell viability assays revealed that an impressive 90.5 ± 0.07% of cells remained viable after 48 hours of culture on poly(butanetetrol fumarate) matrices. This showcases the material's remarkable potential to support cellular growth and viability, crucial factors in tissue engineering (Figure 6.8).

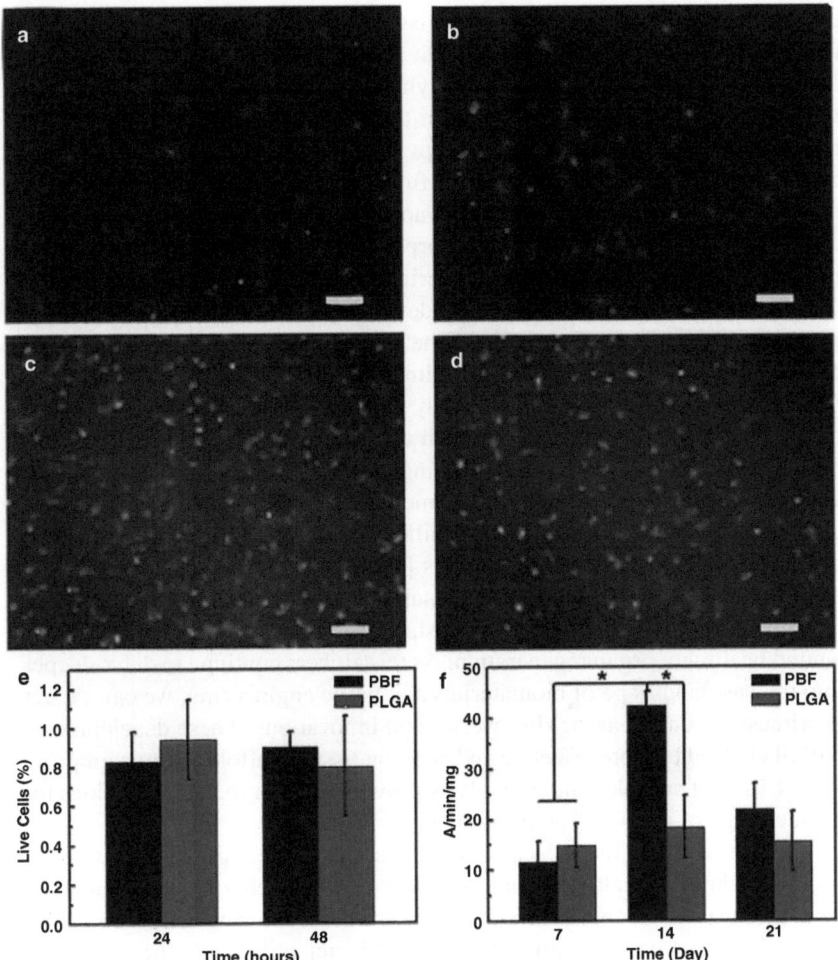

FIGURE 6.8 (a–e) Osteoblasts cultivated on PBF and PLGA were tested for live/dead status and for ALP activity. Fluorescence pictures of osteoblasts cultivated on PBF and PLGA at 24 and 48 hours, respectively. (e) At 24 and 48 hours, the proportion of live cells on both polymers. (f) Assay for alkaline phosphatase activity. Osteoblasts cultivated on PBF and PLGA exhibiting ALP activity (magnification 40x, scale bar 100 m). Reproduced with permission from [21], copyright reserved Royal Society of Chemistry 2019.

What's more, experiments delving into the APA of osteoblasts cultured on the poly(butanetetrol fumarate) matrix illuminated intriguing results. APA exhibited a significant increase from day 7 to day 14, attributable to the presence of excess hydroxyl groups within the polymer structure. This offers exciting prospects for enhancing bone tissue regeneration and osteoblast function, critical in the context of bone repair and regeneration. The tunable nature of the poly(butanetetrol fumarate) polymer adds another layer of versatility to its application [21]. Researchers can tailor its properties, for instance, by incorporating pendant hydroxyl groups, thereby introducing an additional dimension of functionalization. This functionality holds great promise for immobilization and controlled release applications, notably in the controlled delivery of growth factors like bone morphogenetic protein, further enhancing its utility in the realm of tissue engineering and regenerative medicine [21].

The future of tissue scaffolds is undeniably promising and poised for continued growth and innovation. One of the key drivers of this bright future is the ongoing evolution of materials and technology in the field of tissue engineering. These advancements are constantly pushing the boundaries of what can be achieved in the realm of tissue repair and regeneration. Solvent-responsive SMPs stand out as a particularly exciting area of development. Their unique ability to adapt and respond to environmental cues, such as changes in solvent conditions, opens up a world of possibilities for creating more advanced and patient-centric tissue scaffold solutions [22,23]. These SMPs can mimic the dynamic behaviors of living tissues, making them exceptionally well-suited for applications where tissues are constantly evolving and adapting, such as wound healing or organ regeneration. As researchers continue to delve deeper into the vast landscape of biomaterials and tissue engineering, we can expect to witness groundbreaking discoveries and innovations. These developments will likely lead to more effective and efficient tissue scaffold designs, improving the lives of countless individuals by providing better treatment options for a wide range of medical conditions [23].

In the field of tissue scaffold innovation, there's great potential for improving human health and quality of life. As new technologies and materials continue to advance, we envision a future where repairing and regenerating tissues becomes easier, more efficient, and better tailored to the complexities of the human body. This progress promises to bring tangible benefits to people worldwide, offering optimism and healing in the fight against various health issues.

6.3 APPLICATION IN OCCLUSION DEVICES

The utilization of solvent-responsive shape memory effects (SMEs) in occlusion devices represents a highly promising and intriguing area of research, especially within the realm of medical procedures. The potential applications and impact of solvent-responsive SMEs in occlusion devices are substantial, with a particular focus on enhancing the outcomes of medical interventions. The success and practicality of these solvent-responsive SMEs are closely tied to a crucial factor: the speed at which the shape recovery takes place. This factor assumes paramount importance, especially in the context of surgical procedures where time can be of the essence. Much like their heating-responsive SME counterparts, solvent-activated SMEs exhibit a strong reliance on temperature conditions for their effective operation. Temperature plays a pivotal role in determining the rate at which the shape recovery process unfolds. This dependence on temperature introduces a dynamic aspect to the application of solvent-responsive SMEs, wherein environmental conditions and the choice of solvent can significantly influence the device's performance.

For medical practitioners and researchers alike, achieving a balance between the desired shape recovery speed and the environmental conditions is essential. Ideally, the solvent-responsive SME should be able to enact rapid shape recovery, aligning with the urgency often associated with medical procedures. The challenge lies in achieving this expedited recovery while ensuring that the device remains safe and reliable for use in medical applications.

Traditionally, SMP foams have been the subject of extensive research as they offer considerable advantages when used as embolic devices for stabilizing sidewall aneurysms and vascular abnormalities in porcine models [24]. These investigations have not only confirmed the biocompatibility of SMP foams but have also highlighted their potential for clinical applications [24,25]. The studies revealed a significant infiltration of connective tissue throughout the implant, resulting in complete and stable occlusion of treated aneurysms. This process of connective tissue deposition and scar formation is crucial in preventing recanalization, a phenomenon that poses significant risks [26,27].

The unique design of SMP foams is aimed at expediting the maturation of healing processes. These foams provide a scaffold morphology that readily supports the initial clotting of blood within the implant. Over time, this clot is gradually replaced by mature connective tissue. By reducing the time required for mature healing, the risk of recanalization is substantially minimized. This, in turn, leads to a decreased necessity for follow-up imaging, resulting in reduced overall treatment costs [27].

One of the standout features of SMP foams is their ability to be stored in a compressed state and then rapidly expand to occupy significant volumes when they come into contact with circulating blood. This unique shape memory property makes them exceptionally well-suited for minimally invasive medical devices that require low friction during catheter delivery. Despite their compact initial size, SMP foams can expand up to ten times their

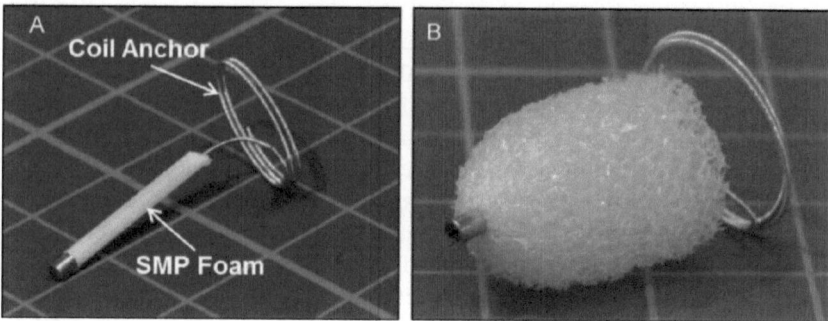

FIGURE 6.9   Image of the crimped (A) and expanded (B) embodiment of the SMP peripheral occlusion device investigated within this study. The device consists of a distal platinum alloy coil anchor and a proximal length of SMP foam that is crimped for delivery through a guide catheter and subsequently undergoes up to 100X volume expansion to fill large volumes upon deployment. Reproduced with permission from [24], copyright reserved Elsevier 2016.

crimped diameter to efficiently block vessels, providing rapid and effective occlusion with just a single device (Figure 6.9) [28].

The potential applicability of solvent-responsive SMEs in occlusion devices is contingent upon the requisite speed of shape recovery, a critical determinant in surgical procedures. In a manner analogous to heating-responsive SME, the effectiveness of solvent-activated SME is intricately tied to the recovery temperature, a topic previously addressed. This particular characteristic endows the system with an additional advantage concerning its practical applications, consequently broadening the spectrum of potential applications for this technology.

With the advent of technology, Wong et al. developed a shape memory occluding device consisting of a composite of a radio-opaque filler and a poly (d lactide-co-glycolide) (PLGA) blend, which was coated with a crosslinked poly (ethylene glycol) diacrylate (PEGDA) hydrogel. The bioabsorbable radioopaque embolic plug, founded on the water-triggered shape memory of a composite material comprising PLGA-PEGDA hydrogel, has been effectively engineered and subjected to comprehensive evaluation, encompassing crucial metrics of its suitability as an embolic agent. These evaluations have primarily centered around its performance in terms of both occlusion efficiency and biodegradation, particularly through in vitro experimentation [29].

Furthermore, in vivo assessments involving the utilization of these embolic plugs in a rabbit embolization model have been conducted. The findings from these studies have revealed several significant outcomes. Notably, the prototypes have demonstrated visibility under fluoroscopy, thereby ensuring their traceability during medical procedures. Moreover, they have exhibited a remarkable capacity for inducing complete vascular occlusion within a remarkably short timeframe, consistently achieving this outcome in less than two minutes in all cases studied [29].

Investigating the mechanism of solvent responsiveness, the biodegradable SMP in this system [29] has a dual purpose: first, it acts as a "carrier" or scaffold for the hydrogel, and second, it offers radio-opacity to allow viewing of the device under x-ray imaging. Furthermore, the hydrogel component creates a driving force for the device's water-induced actuation, resulting in mechanical anchoring of the plug and total occlusion of the blood vessel. Using these materials, a prototype embolic plug was created and designed to have shape memory capabilities via thermal deformation into a temporary shape at 70°C (Figure 6.10) [29].

In the context of in vivo applications, the rate of embolization (or occlusion) is as important as the level of total occlusion, a measure known as "embolization efficiency." This efficiency was tested in vitro, with a custom-designed flow model simulating blood flow within an artery. As shown in Figure 6.10, when the created prototype is deployed through a 4-F catheter (at 0 seconds), water molecules begin diffusing into the system, kicking off the water-triggered recovery process of the hydrogel covering. Following that, the PLGA core begins to recover and buckle until its form recovery exceeds the resistance of the PEG hydrogel coating. This sequence of events leads to the anchoring of the device to the vessel wall within 16 seconds of deployment, as evidenced by a significant reduction in the flow rate depicted [29]. At this juncture, the device becomes mechanically locked and anchored at the intended site, resulting in complete occlusion facilitated by the swelling of the hydrogel, which occurs by 120 seconds. This ultimately culminates in a halt at 120 seconds, signifying the attainment of complete "embolization" or occlusion of the flow channel [29].

These results collectively signify that the developed embolic plug holds substantial promise as a biocompatible and biodegradable embolic agent suitable for temporary embolization. While these findings are indeed promising, it is worth noting that further investigations may be warranted to attain a comprehensive understanding of the in vivo degradation profile and the subsequent recanalization rate of the embolized artery. Additionally, it would be valuable to delve into the tissue response to temporary occlusion facilitated by the embolic plug. Expanding the evaluation to encompass additional time points would serve to enhance the comprehensiveness of these assessments and provide a more detailed perspective on the long-term performance and safety of the embolic plug.

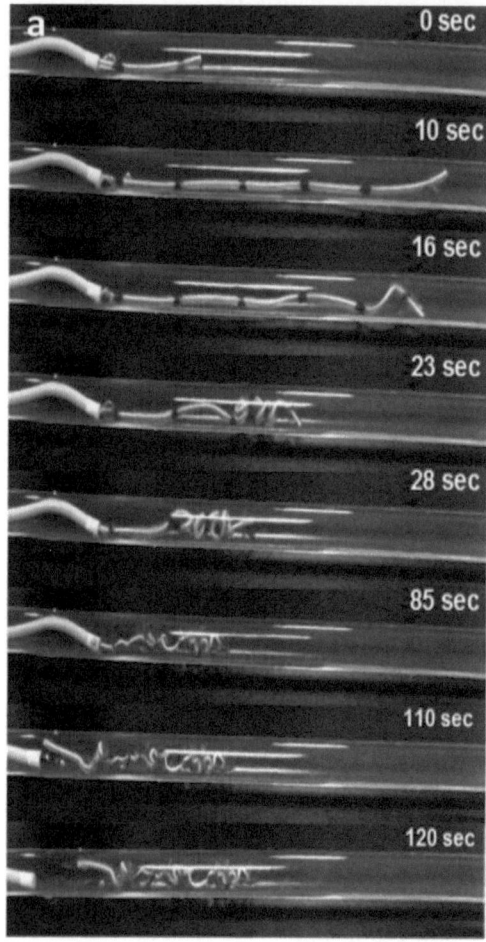

FIGURE 6.10   (a) In vitro embolization and responsiveness by the developed embolic plug. Reproduced with permission from [29], copyright reserved Elsevier 2016.

6.4 APPLICATION IN DRUG DELIVERY DEVICES

SMPs have garnered significant attention in the realm of biomedical applications, particularly in scenarios where controlled drug release and reduced inflammation responses are essential, such as in drug-eluting stents. This formalized discussion outlines the pioneering research efforts in this field, showcasing how researchers have harnessed SMP technology for drug incorporation and release.

Building upon this foundation, Jaworska et al. advanced the field by integrating antirestenotic drugs into SMP stents. Their groundbreaking work demonstrated sustained drug release, facilitated by the gradual degradation properties inherent to SMP matrices. Incorporating an antirestenotic drug into a biodegradable SMP stent appears to be a promising solution due to its potential to combine mechanical support with controlled drug elution. In the study at hand, sirolimus was introduced into poly(l-lactide-co-glycolide-co-trimethylene carbonate) using the injection molding method, and its impact on drug incorporation was thoroughly examined. This particular terpolymer was selected for the investigation because of its favorable characteristics, including biodegradability, biocompatibility, and shape memory properties (at 37°C, with a recovery ratio (R_r) of 100%.) [30]. Similar controlled release mechanism was also observed in the SMP systems developed by Xiao et al. (crosslinked poly(ε-caprolactone)/poly(sebacic anhydride)) [31] and by Kashif et al. (poly(ε-caprolactone)/polyhedral oligomeric silsequioxane nanocomposites) [32].

Correia and Mano made a significant contribution to the field by pioneering the design of a chitosan-based SMP scaffold [20]. Their innovative approach involved incorporating drugs into swelled polymer matrices, and subsequent drying processes yielded a distinctive drug release profile. This profile exhibited rapid drug release within the first two hours of wetting, followed by a substantially slower release rate.

Their work exemplifies the remarkable potential of SMPs in the realm of biomedical applications. These materials offer a versatile platform for addressing critical requirements in the field, including precise control over drug release and compatibility with biological systems. The strategic integration of pharmaceutical agents into SMP matrices, coupled with the inherent shape memory properties of these materials, opens up a compelling avenue for the development of advanced medical devices and therapeutic systems. This pioneering research not only advances the understanding of SMPs but also holds promise for improving patient care and medical treatment. It underscores the importance of interdisciplinary approaches that combine materials science, engineering, and biomedicine to address complex healthcare challenges. The ability to fine-tune drug release profiles in a controlled manner can have a profound impact on the efficacy and safety of medical treatments, making SMPs a valuable tool in the development of next-generation biomedical devices and therapies [20].

Although nascent, in a pioneering breakthrough, researchers have introduced a groundbreaking concept—water-responsive shape memory poly(vinyl alcohol) (SM-PVA) with a programmable shape recovery process. This innovative approach leverages a wettability-contrast strategy to enable the precise definition of regional water-responsive properties within SM-PVA, expanding its versatility and functionality for biomedical applications and beyond, especially in the sector of proactive drug delivery [33]. The core of this innovation involves the deposition of hexamethyldisilazane (HMDS)-treated SiO_2 nanoparticles onto the surface of SM-PVA (Figure 6.11). These nanoparticles are applied with varying coating weights, resulting in a strategic contrast in surface wettability across the material. This deliberate variation in wettability induces distinct changes in the water absorption behavior of SM-PVA. Importantly, these alterations in water absorption can be accurately described using a pseudo-first-order kinetic model [33].

What sets this research apart is the ability to program and control the shape recovery process of water-responsive SM-PVA. By orchestrating the sequence of various coated regions with different SiO_2 coating weights or by increasing the SiO_2-coated surface area, researchers have achieved a programmable multistep shape recovery process. This breakthrough holds immense promise for creating highly adaptable and precisely controlled shape memory materials (Figure 6.11).

The significance of this advancement is further underscored by the development of two proof-of-concept drug delivery devices, each featuring distinct three-dimensional structures and precisely controlled actuation mechanisms. These devices are constructed using the programmable water-responsive SM-PVA and serve as tangible examples of their potential in the biomedical field.

In a broader context, the emergence of water-responsive SMPs, as illustrated by the innovative methodology involving SM-PVA with programmable shape recovery, represents a seminal breakthrough, particularly within the sphere of biomedical applications. This pioneering approach holds the promise of unlocking a multitude of opportunities with the capacity to fundamentally transform the landscape of healthcare and medicine. The biomedical domain, characterized by its diverse array of fields, stands to benefit significantly from the distinctive properties and capabilities inherent in these polymers.

Biomedical applications encompass a wide spectrum of disciplines, and the inherent adaptability of water-responsive SM-PVA introduces a realm of intriguing prospects spanning this spectrum. Among these, drug delivery emerges as a particularly promising frontier, where the precise modulation of drug release assumes paramount importance. Leveraging the programmable shape recovery process, these polymers can be ingeniously employed to devise intelligent drug delivery systems capable of administering medications with unprecedented precision. This technological advancement holds the potential to augment therapeutic effectiveness while mitigating the occurrence of undesirable side effects.

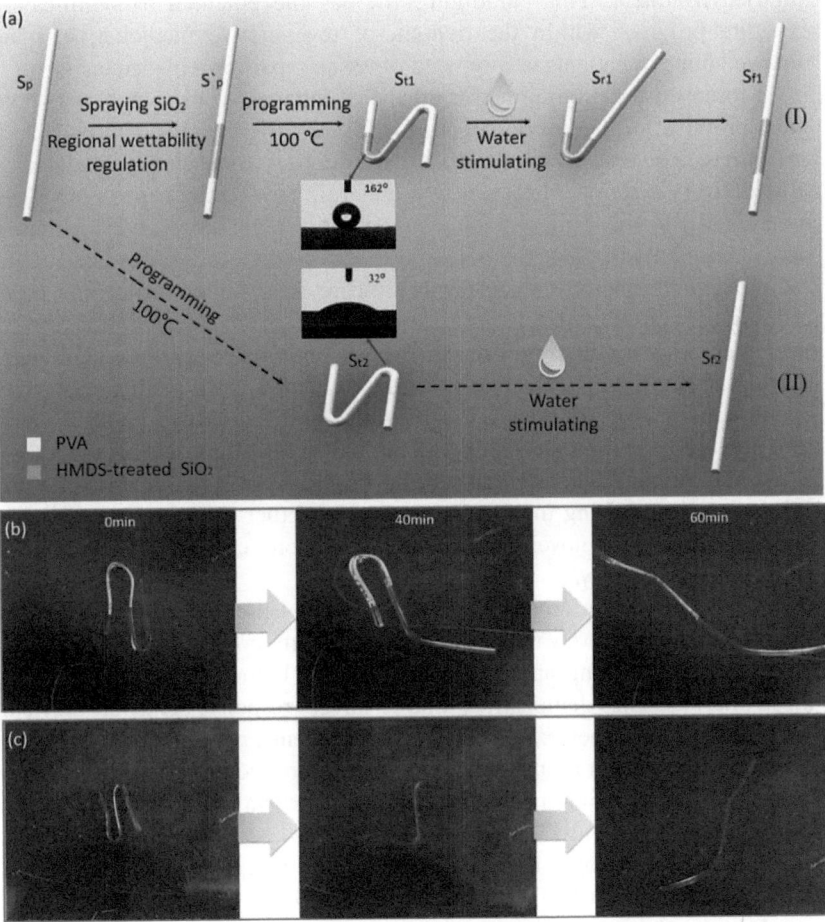

FIGURE 6.11 (a) Schematic appearance the directing and programming cycle of water-responsive SM-PVAs and their entire shape recuperation process in water. Advanced photos show the shape recuperation cycles of (b) SM-PVA with a HMDS-treated SiO_2 nanoparticle layer and (c) unadulterated SM-PVA. Note that the pictures from left to right in boards b and c address the transitory shape, halfway shape, and unique shape. Reproduced with permission from [33], copyright reserved American Chemical Society 2017.

Concurrently, the field of tissue engineering stands poised on the precipice of transformation. The pivotal role played by biocompatible scaffolds in facilitating tissue regeneration and wound healing is undeniable. The versatility of water-responsive SM-PVA empowers the creation of scaffolds endowed with adjustable properties that closely emulate the native tissue microenvironment. This paradigm shift has the potential to significantly expedite progress within the domain of regenerative medicine, offering renewed hope to patients in dire need of tissue repair or replacement.

Moreover, the programmable attributes intrinsic to these polymers hold great promise for the development of intelligent implantable devices. These encompass a diverse array of applications, ranging from sensors to advanced drug delivery systems. These devices, underpinned by their capacity to adapt dynamically to changing physiological conditions, not only serve to enhance patient care but also have the potential to curtail the need for invasive medical procedures, thereby rendering healthcare interventions safer and more efficacious.

Integrating multi-stimuli responsiveness into materials holds significant promise, especially in fields like biomedicine. Through the method of interfacial polymerization, we've developed a range of oil-in-water core-shell structure polyurethane microcapsules with multi-stimuli-responsive behavior [34]. These microcapsules boast adjustable surface morphology and a specific carrying capacity, making them stand out among other capsules and particles. Notably, they exhibit novel shape memory functions, enhancing their controllability and versatility.

What sets these microcapsules apart is their release temperature of 35.4°C, which is lower than body temperature. This feature presents a distinct advantage when considering applications within the human body. Furthermore, these microcapsules demonstrate unique solvent response behavior; they can swell and rupture when exposed to organic solvents, releasing their contents. This capability holds promise for precisely controlled drug release, with the analysis of the swelling mechanism providing crucial insights for the development of new systems [34–36].

Beyond these properties, there are other response behaviors of the microcapsules that warrant further investigation and development. Based on these capabilities, multi-stimuli-responsive microcapsules hold immense potential in biomedicine. They could revolutionize applications such as drug release and self-healing, offering innovative solutions to pressing medical challenges. This underscores the importance of ongoing research and development in this exciting field, paving the way for transformative advancements in healthcare and beyond.

As this pioneering work gains momentum, it carries with it the potential to substantially enhance patient outcomes, mitigate healthcare expenditures, and elevate the overall standard of medical care [37]. The convergence of materials science and medicine stands poised to yield transformative breakthroughs, effectively reshaping the landscape of healthcare and pushing the frontiers of what can be achieved within the realm of biomedical technology.

REFERENCES

1. Hanawa, T. (2009). Materials for metallic stents. *Journal of Artificial Organs*, *12*, 73–79.
2. Watt, A. M., Faragher, I. G., Griffin, T. T., Rieger, N. A., & Maddern, G. J. (2007). Self-expanding metallic stents for relieving malignant colorectal obstruction: A systematic review. *Annals of Surgery*, *246*(1), 24.
3. Basak, S., & Bandyopadhyay, A. (2021). Solvent responsive shape memory polymers-evolution, current status, and future outlook. *Macromolecular Chemistry and Physics*, *222*(19), 2100195.
4. Tamai, H., Igaki, K., Kyo, E., Kosuga, K., Kawashima, A., Matsui, S., ... & Uehata, H. (2000). Initial and 6-month results of biodegradable poly-l-lactic acid coronary stents in humans. *Circulation*, *102*(4), 399–404.
5. Venkatraman, S. S., Tan, L. P., Joso, J. F. D., Boey, Y. C. F., & Wang, X. (2006). Biodegradable stents with elastic memory. *Biomaterials*, *27*(8), 1573–1578.
6. Dallal, H. J., Smith, G. D., Grieve, D. C., Ghosh, S., Penman, I. D., & Palmer, K. R. (2001). A randomized trial of thermal ablative therapy versus expandable metal stents in the palliative treatment of patients with esophageal carcinoma. *Gastrointestinal Endoscopy*, *54*(5), 549–557.
7. Basak, S., & Bandyopadhyay, A. (2022). two-way semicrystalline shape memory elastomers: Development and current research trends. *Advanced Engineering Materials*, *24*(10), 2200257.
8. Chen, M. C., Tsai, H. W., Chang, Y., Lai, W. Y., Mi, F. L., Liu, C. T., ... & Sung, H. W. (2007). Rapidly self-expandable polymeric stents with a shape-memory property. *Biomacromolecules*, *8*(9), 2774–2780
9. Lohrr, J. M., Budig, L., Sagartz, J., Girida, S., Thyagarajan, K., & Tu, R. (1992). Evaluation of two epoxy ether compounds for biocompatible potential. *Artificial Organs*, *16*(6), 630–633.
10. Park, S. A., Lee, S. J., Lim, K. S., Bae, I. H., Lee, J. H., Kim, W. D., ... & Park, J. K. (2015). In vivo evaluation and characterization of a bio-absorbable drug-coated stent fabricated using a 3D-printing system. *Materials Letters*, *141*, 355–358.
11. Dobrzynski, P. I. O. T. R., Sobota, M. I. C. H. A. Ł., Smola, A. N. N. A., Kasperczyk, J. A. N. U. S. Z., Kokot, G. R. Z. E. G. O. R. Z., & Kuś, W. A. C. Ł. A. W. (2016). Bioresorbable self-expanded vascular stents-the preliminary results. ENGINEERING OF BIOMATERIALS 138 (2016) 41] https://bibliotekanauki.pl/articles/284678.pdf
12. Zopf, D. A., Hollister, S. J., Nelson, M. E., Ohye, R. G., & Green, G. E. (2013). Bioresorbable airway splint created with a three-dimensional printer. *New England Journal of Medicine*, *368*(21), 2043–2045.
13. Yeazel, T. R., & Becker, M. L. (2020). Advancing toward 3D printing of bioresorbable shape memory polymer stents. *Biomacromolecules*, *21*(10), 3957–3965.
14. Guo, B., & Ma, P. X. (2014). Synthetic biodegradable functional polymers for tissue engineering: A brief review. *Science China Chemistry*, *57*, 490–500.

15. Thomson, R. C., Shung, A. K., Yaszemski, M. J., & Mikos, A. G. (2000). Polymer scaffold processing. *Principles of Tissue Engineering*, 2, 251–262.
16. Shoichet, M. S. (2010). Polymer scaffolds for biomaterials applications. *Macromolecules*, *43*(2), 581–591.
17. Xiao, R., & Huang, W. M. (2020). Heating/solvent responsive shape-memory polymers for implant biomedical devices in minimally invasive surgery: Current status and challenge. *Macromolecular Bioscience*, *20*(8), 2000108.
18. Hutmacher, D. W. (2001). Scaffold design and fabrication technologies for engineering tissues—state of the art and future perspectives. *Journal of Biomaterials Science, Polymer Edition*, *12*(1), 107–124.
19. Beilvert, A., Chaubet, F., Chaunier, L., Guilois, S., Pavon-Djavid, G., Letourneur, D., ... & Lourdin, D. (2014). Shape-memory starch for resorbable biomedical devices. *Carbohydrate Polymers*, *99*, 242–248.
20. Correia, C. O., & Mano, J. F. (2014). Chitosan scaffolds with a shape memory effect induced by hydration. *Journal of Materials Chemistry B*, *2*(21), 3315–3323.
21. Guo, Y., Lv, Z., Huo, Y., Sun, L., Chen, S., Liu, Z., ... & You, Z. (2019). A biodegradable functional water-responsive shape memory polymer for biomedical applications. *Journal of Materials Chemistry B*, *7*(1), 123–132.
22. Hu, X., He, J., Yong, X., Lu, J., Xiao, J., Liao, Y., ... & Xiong, C. (2020). Biodegradable poly (lactic acid-co-trimethylene carbonate)/chitosan microsphere scaffold with shape-memory effect for bone tissue engineering. *Colloids and Surfaces B: Biointerfaces*, *195*, 111218.
23. Saghati, S., Rahbarghazi, R., Fathi Karkan, S., Nazifkerdar, S., Khoshfetrat, A. B., & Tayefi Nasrabadi, H. (2022). Shape memory polymers in osteochondral tissue engineering. *Journal of Research in Clinical Medicine*, *10*, 30.
24. Landsman, T. L., Bush, R. L., Glowczwski, A., Horn, J., Jessen, S. L., Ungchusri, E., ... & Maitland, D. J. (2016). Design and verification of a shape memory polymer peripheral occlusion device. *Journal of the Mechanical Behavior of Biomedical Materials*, *63*, 195–206.
25. Rodriguez, J. N., Clubb, F. J., Wilson, T. S., Miller, M. W., Fossum, T. W., Hartman, J., ... & Maitland, D. J. (2014). In vivo response to an implanted shape memory polyurethane foam in a porcine aneurysm model. *Journal of Biomedical Materials Research Part A*, *102*(5), 1231–1242.
26. Rodriguez, J. N., Miller, M. W., Boyle, A., Horn, J., Yang, C. K., Wilson, T. S., ... & Maitland, D. J. (2014). Reticulation of low density shape memory polymer foam with an in vivo demonstration of vascular occlusion. *Journal of the Mechanical Behavior of Biomedical Materials*, *40*, 102–114.
27. Bavinzski, G., Talazoglu, V., Killer, M., Richling, B., Gruber, A., Gross, C. E., & Plenk, H. (1999). Gross and microscopic histopathological findings in aneurysms of the human brain treated with Guglielmi detachable coils. *Journal of neurosurgery*, *91*(2), 284–293.
28. Singhal, P., Rodriguez, J. N., Small, W., Eagleston, S., Van de Water, J., Maitland, D. J., & Wilson, T. S. (2012). Ultra low density and highly cross-linked biocompatible shape memory polyurethane foams. *Journal of Polymer Science Part B: Polymer Physics*, *50*(10), 724–737.

29. Wong, Y. S., Salvekar, A. V., Da Zhuang, K., Liu, H., Birch, W. R., Tay, K. H., ... & Venkatraman, S. S. (2016). Bioabsorbable radiopaque water-responsive shape memory embolization plug for temporary vascular occlusion. *Biomaterials*, *102*, 98–106.

30. Jaworska, J., Jelonek, K., Sobota, M., Kasperczyk, J., Dobrzynski, P., Musial-Kulik, M., ... & Jarzabek, B. (2015). Shape-memory bioresorbable terpolymer composite with antirestenotic drug. *Journal of Applied Polymer Science*, *132*(17), 41902.

31. Xiao, Y., Zhou, S., Wang, L., Zheng, X., & Gong, T. (2010). Crosslinked poly (ε-caprolactone)/poly (sebacic anhydride) composites combining biodegradation, controlled drug release and shape memory effect. *Composites Part B: Engineering*, *41*(7), 537–542.

32. Kashif, M., Yun, B. M., Lee, K. S., & Chang, Y. W. (2016). Biodegradable shape-memory poly (ε-caprolactone)/polyhedral oligomeric silsequioxane nanocomposites: Sustained drug release and hydrolytic degradation. *Materials Letters*, *166*, 125–128.

33. Fang, Z., Kuang, Y., Zhou, P., Ming, S., Zhu, P., Liu, Y., ... & Chen, G. (2017). Programmable shape recovery process of water-responsive shape-memory poly (vinyl alcohol) by wettability contrast strategy. *ACS Applied Materials & Interfaces*, *9*(6), 5495–5502.

34. Zhang, F., Wang, L., Geng, Q., Liu, Y., Leng, J., & Smoukov, S. K. (2023). Adjustable volume and loading release of shape memory polymer microcapsules. *International Journal of Smart and Nano Materials*, *14*(1), 77–89.

35. Basak, S. (2024). Is grafting crystals the new art of making conventional elastomers smart?. *The Canadian Journal of Chemical Engineering*, 102(7), 2432–2442.

36. Basak, S. (2020). The age of multistimuli-responsive nanogels: The finest evolved nano delivery system in biomedical sciences. *Biotechnology and Bioprocess Engineering*, *25*(5), 655–669.

37. Delaey, J., Dubruel, P., & Van Vlierberghe, S. (2020). Shape-memory polymers for biomedical applications. *Advanced Functional Materials*, *30*(44), 1909047.

Exploring the Structure-Property Relationships of Solvent-Responsive SMPs

7

Exploring the structure-property relationships of solvent-responsive SMPs involves a comprehensive investigation into how the chemical composition, molecular architecture, and processing conditions of these materials influence their behavior in different solvent environments [1,2]. The polymer composition plays a crucial role, with the choice of monomers impacting the responsiveness of SMPs to solvents [1]. For instance, incorporating hydrophilic or hydrophobic groups can influence the polymer's affinity toward specific solvents. The crosslinking density within the polymer network is another key parameter affecting solvent interaction; higher crosslinking can decrease solvent permeability and alter swelling behavior [1–4].

Furthermore, understanding the polymer's microstructure and morphology is essential. Factors such as crystallinity, phase separation, and chain mobility influence how the polymer swells or contracts in response to solvent exposure [4]. The architecture of the polymer network, whether linear or branched, also impacts solvent-induced shape changes. Solvent interaction and swelling behavior are dependent on the polarity of the solvent. Evaluating

DOI: 10.1201/9781003593805-7

the Flory-Huggins (FH) interaction parameters can provide insights into polymer-solvent miscibility and swelling kinetics [4].

To investigate these relationships, various characterization techniques are employed. Swelling studies using gravimetry or dimensional measurements offer quantitative data on solvent uptake and release. Spectroscopic analysis techniques like FTIR, NMR, or Raman spectroscopy reveal molecular interactions occurring during solvent exposure. Microscopy, such as SEM or AFM, allows visualization of changes in polymer morphology induced by solvents.

Thermal and mechanical properties are also significant. The glass transition temperature (T_g) of the SMP correlates with its solvent responsiveness and shape memory effect (SME). Mechanical testing helps evaluate changes in material properties upon exposure to solvents, which is crucial for assessing the material's performance in practical applications.

Ultimately, a systematic experimental approach involving design of experiments (DOE) and analytical modeling is employed to uncover predictive relationships between polymer structure and solvent-responsive properties [5]. This research not only advances fundamental knowledge but also guides the design and development of solvent-responsive SMPs tailored for specific applications ranging from biomedical devices to smart textiles and sensors.

Figure 7.1a illustrates the typical dynamic behavior of an amorphous thermoset, showcasing its response to changes in temperature and the associated storage modulus. In amorphous shape memory polymers (SMPs), such as thermosets, the storage modulus undergoes a substantial decrease of two to three orders of magnitude within the glass transition region [6–8]. This transition is characterized by a distinctive rubbery plateau, indicating a stable molecular structure within this temperature range. The presence of the rubbery plateau suggests that the thermoset maintains its shape and structural integrity even as it transitions through the glass transition temperature (T_g) [9].

On the other hand, Figure 7.1b demonstrates the dynamic response of an amorphous thermoplastic poly(ethylene terephthalate)-glycol (PETG) to temperature variations. Unlike thermosets, amorphous thermoplastics like PETG exhibit a continuous decrease in modulus with increasing temperature, reflecting their inherent instability at higher temperatures [10]. This unique property of amorphous thermoplastics enables them to undergo shape changes permanently when subjected to elevated temperatures, a characteristic that makes them suitable for applications such as filament-based 3D printing using fused deposition modeling (FDM).

The study of glass transition behaviors in these SMPs can be further elucidated by measuring changes in volume or length during thermal cycling experiments. These measurements provide valuable insights into how the molecular structure and interactions within the polymer matrix respond to

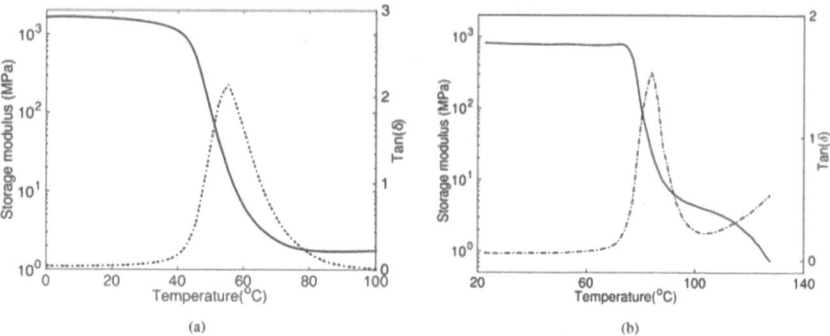

FIGURE 7.1   Typical DMA results of (a) amorphous acrylate-based SMP and (b) amorphous thermoplastic PETG. Reprinted with permission from [6], Copyright reserved Wiley 2020.

temperature variations, impacting the material's mechanical properties and shape memory capabilities. By understanding these dynamic behaviors, researchers can optimize the design and processing of SMPs for specific applications that require tailored thermal and mechanical properties, including shape memory functionality and thermal stability during processing like 3D printing [8–10].

In the context of applications like minimally invasive surgery, it is crucial for SMP-based devices to endure repetitive deformations. Therefore, conducting a range of mechanical tests that involve large deformations becomes essential to assess the material's performance. These tests typically involve subjecting the SMPs to uniaxial tension and compression modes while varying parameters such as deformation temperature and strain rate [6].

Figure 7.2a provides insights into the stress response of amorphous PETG under uniaxial compression across its glass transition region. Above the glass transition temperature, these polymers exhibit viscoelastic behavior, meaning they demonstrate both viscous (flow) and elastic (recovery) properties under stress. Conversely, below T_g, the polymers display a viscoplastic response characterized by yielding (a point where the material permanently deforms), strain softening (a decrease in stiffness with increasing strain), and strain hardening (an increase in stiffness after yielding) under significant strain.

It is noteworthy that the stress response of these materials is also influenced by the strain rate; higher rates of deformation result in increased stress levels. Additionally, deforming the SMPs in their glassy state (below T_g) requires significantly more force than deforming them in their rubbery state (above T_g), highlighting the distinct mechanical behavior across the glass transition temperature.

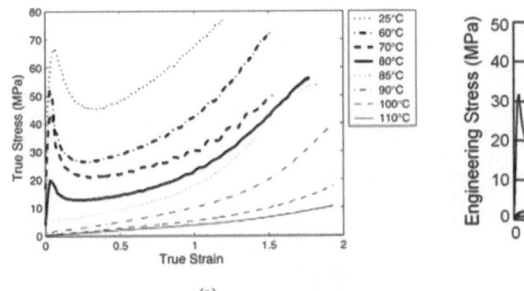
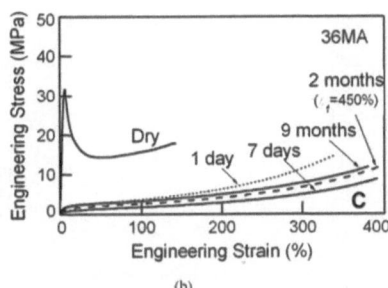

(a)   (b)

FIGURE 7.2   (a) The temperature-dependent stress response in uniaxial compression of PETG and (b) the stress response of (meth)acrylate-based networks immersed in phosphate buffer saline (PBS) for different amounts of time. Reprinted with permission from [6], Copyright reserved Wiley 2020.

Understanding these mechanical responses is crucial for designing SMP-based devices that can withstand the demands of practical applications like minimally invasive surgery, where repeated and controlled deformations are essential. By characterizing the material's behavior under different loading conditions and temperatures, engineers and researchers can optimize the design and performance of SMPs to ensure reliability and functionality in specific operational environments.

Similarly, the stress response of semicrystalline polymers exhibits similar dependencies on temperature and strain rate as observed in amorphous polymers. Additionally, the presence of solvents significantly impacts the stress response of these polymers. When solvents diffuse into the polymer matrix, there is a notable transition in the material's mechanical behavior. Initially, the polymer may exhibit a stiff viscoplastic response [6]. However, as solvent penetration increases, the material's response shifts toward a softer, more viscoelastic behavior. This transition is illustrated in Figure 7.2b, showcasing the evolution of mechanical properties due to solvent exposure.

In practical applications, SMPs are essential for fulfilling specific mechanical requirements tailored to diverse needs. Figures 7.3 and 7.4 provide valuable insights into how the glass transition temperature (T_g) correlates with mechanical properties like Young's modulus and yield strength across different types of polymers [6].

Figure 7.3 illustrates this correlation for amorphous polymers, showcasing transition temperatures that can exceed 260°C. This range of T_g values reflects the varying thermal stability of these polymers, which is crucial for applications requiring high-temperature resistance. Additionally, the Young's modulus displayed in Figure 7.3 spans from as low as 10 MPa to several

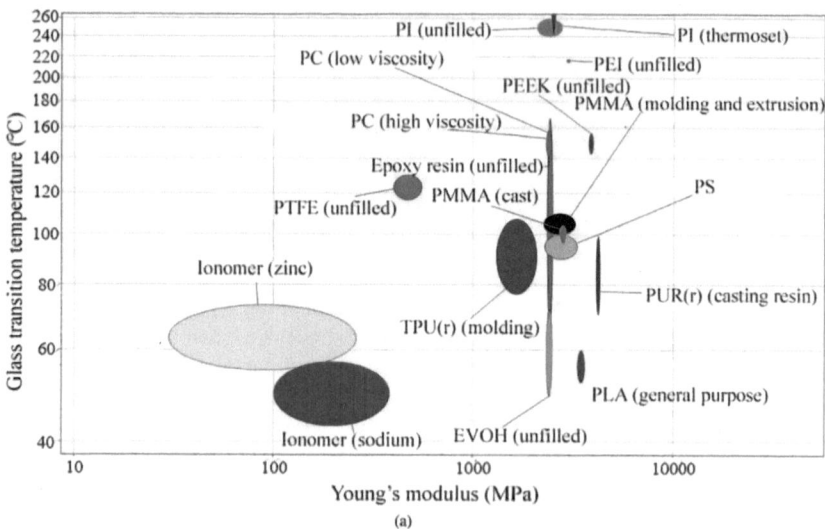

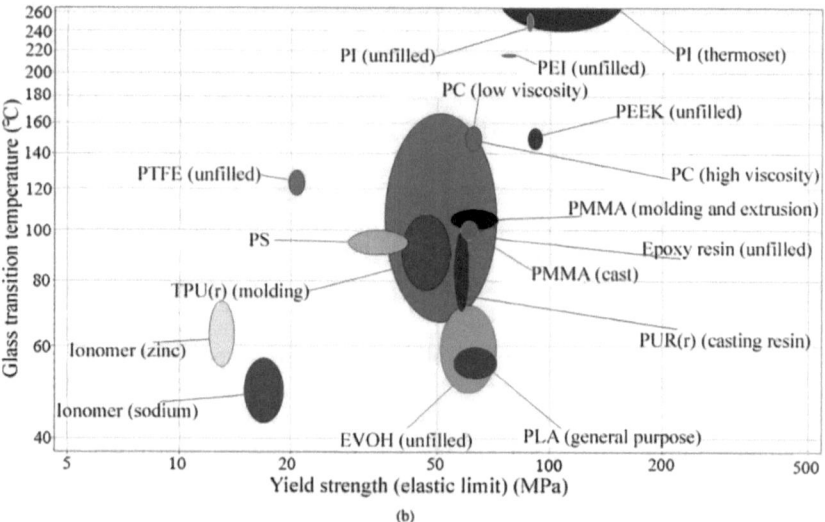

FIGURE 7.3 T_g as a function of (a) Young's modulus and (b) yield strength of typical engineering polymers. Reprinted with permission from [6], Copyright reserved Wiley 2020.

thousand MPa among different amorphous polymers. This broad spectrum of stiffness allows for the selection of SMPs with tailored flexibility or rigidity, depending on the specific application requirements.

Similarly, Figure 7.4 presents analogous data for semicrystalline polymers, demonstrating even higher transition temperatures that can reach up

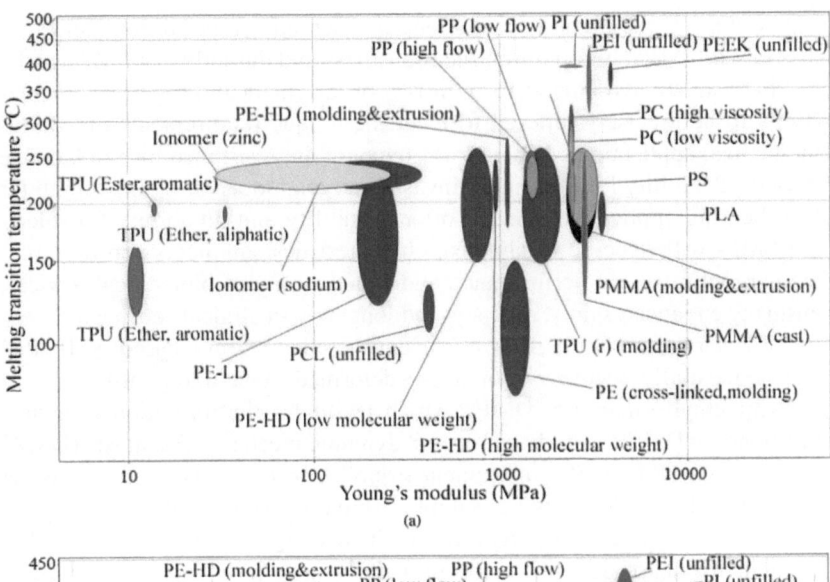

(a)

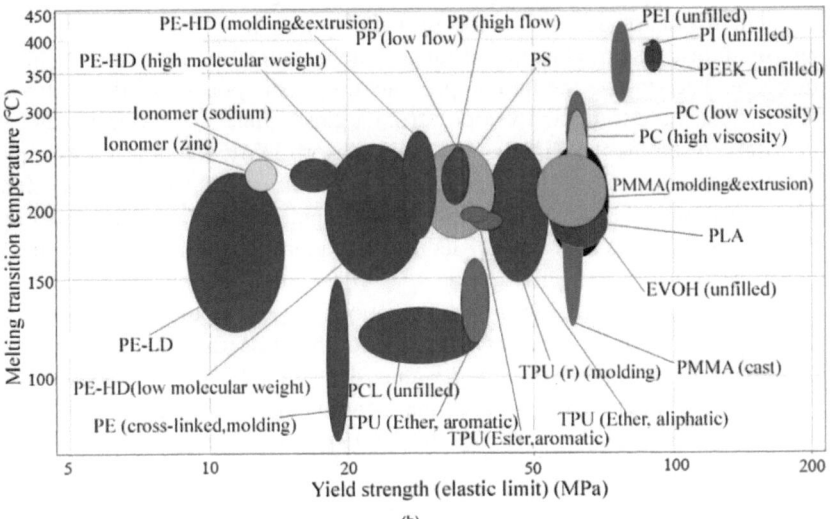

(b)

FIGURE 7.4 Melting transition temperature (T_m) as a function of (a) Young's modulus and (b) yield strength of typical engineering polymers. Reprinted with permission from [6], Copyright reserved Wiley 2020.

to 400°C. The substantial thermal stability of semicrystalline SMPs makes them suitable for demanding environments where extreme temperatures are encountered. The range of Young's modulus observed in semicrystalline polymers also offers significant variability, allowing for the customization of SMPs with specific mechanical properties [6].

Moreover, the highest yield strength observed across all polymer types exceeds 100 MPa, highlighting the robustness and durability of SMPs under mechanical stress. This diverse array of mechanical properties enables SMPs to be precisely tailored to meet the unique requirements of various biomedical applications. Whether it's temperature resistance for implantable devices, flexibility for minimally invasive surgical tools, or high strength for load-bearing applications, SMPs offer versatility and reliability. By selecting SMPs with specific mechanical characteristics, engineers and researchers can optimize the performance and functionality of biomedical devices, ensuring enhanced safety, efficacy, and longevity in clinical settings.

To elaborate on this, Du et al. developed a styrene-based SMP that can sequentially recover from a pre-deformed state upon immersion in N,N-dimethylformamide (DMF), which facilitates the formation of hydrogen bonding [11]. The study conducted dynamic mechanical analysis (DMA) tests using a DMA Q800 instrument from TA Instruments, with a constant frequency of 1 Hz. Rectangular samples were immersed in DMF for different durations at room temperature, followed by heating at a rate of 5°C/min [11].

The results of the DMA tests provide insights into the changes in storage modulus, loss modulus, and tangent delta (tan δ) as functions of temperature. The storage modulus represents the elastic portion of the material and indicates the transition velocity from a glassy state to a rubbery state. It is observed that as the samples gradually absorb DMF solution, the storage modulus decreases from 1,475 MPa (at 0 min immersion) to 604 MPa (after 120 min immersion) at 25°C. The transition temperature, as determined by the storage modulus curves, also decreases gradually with increasing immersion time [11].

Tangent delta (tan δ), defined as the ratio of the loss modulus to the storage modulus, is used as an alternative measure of the glass transition temperature (T_g). According to the results, the T_g values determined from the peaks of tangent delta curves decrease as the immersion time increases. Specifically, T_g is measured as 84.29°C, 74.04°C, 65.30°C, 60.72°C, and 55.05°C for immersion times of 0, 10, 30, 60, and 120 minutes, respectively. The decreasing T_g values and the shift in tan δ peaks indicate changes in the polymer's viscoelastic behavior due to DMF absorption [11].

The DMA results suggest that the mechanical properties of the styrene-based SMP are adversely affected by immersion in DMF due to hydrogen bonding formation. The bonding between polymer and solvent molecules increases the flexibility of the polymeric chains, which in turn negatively impacts the overall mechanical properties of the polymer. This phenomenon aligns with principles from the physics of polymers, highlighting the intricate relationship between molecular interactions, solvent absorption, and material behavior.

In addition to understanding the structure-property relationships of polymers, it is crucial to recognize how these relationships closely guide the shape recovery process of polymers, particularly in the context of shape memory polyurethane foam volume recovery, as highlighted in this study [12]. Swelling and SMEs are pivotal factors influencing SMP behavior. Previous research on solvent-stimulated actuation has indicated that solvent swelling within the polymer matrix alters internal energy and decreases relaxation time [12].

Studies conducted by Boyle et al. revealed significant findings regarding the behavior of foam compositions submerged in 100% solutions of DMSO (dimethyl sulfoxide) and EtOH (ethanol) [12]. All foam compositions exhibited swelling beyond their original volumes during immersion, with similar rates of volume ratio increase observed across compositions during both swelling and volume recovery experiments. However, exposure to EtOH led to an anticipated decrease in relaxation time and Tg (tan δ_{max}) values below 37°C for all foam compositions. Conversely, DMSO exposure resulted in polymer swelling but minimal to no relaxation observed in DMA kinetic experiments [12].

This distinction suggests differing mechanisms through which DMSO and EtOH influence volume recovery in SMPs. During swelling, solvent penetration into the polymer matrix separates polymer chains, increasing overall volume and facilitating viscous migration between the polymer network and solvent. Conversely, during shape recovery, heating the polymer above its transition temperature (T_{trans}) increases chain mobility, allowing entropic forces to orient polymer chains from the organized state of the temporary shape back to the disorganized state of the original shape.

What we understand is that the study underscores that DMSO exposure primarily induces volume change through solvent swelling, which separates polymer chains and increases volume, while stimulation of the conformational change during polymer chain orientation expected during shape recovery is less pronounced. On the other hand, EtOH exposure was observed to cause both volume change from swelling and relaxation during shape recovery, resulting in rapid volume recovery driven by both swelling-induced volume change and expected chain relaxation. The mechanism and effectiveness of solvent-stimulated actuation in SMP systems heavily rely on the molecular interactions between the solvent and the polymer backbone. In the context of polyurethane-based SMP foams, it was observed that ethanol (EtOH) acted as a much more effective plasticizer than dimethyl sulfoxide (DMSO) and water. This enhanced effectiveness can be attributed to two primary factors:

Firstly, EtOH demonstrates a higher capability to penetrate the SMP and plasticize the polymer backbone. Studies by Lu et al. showed that immersion in EtOH over time led to a decrease in the glass transition temperature (Tg) of polyurethanes due to hydrogen bonding interactions between the solvent and the urethane linkages. This interaction facilitates increased mobility of the polymer chains, enhancing the plasticization effect [13].

Secondly, the availability of isocyanate species for plasticization and mobility plays a crucial role. The structure of EtOH allows for effective interactions with the polymer backbone [12]. The hydroxyl (OH) functionality in EtOH readily interacts with the urethane linkages, while the carbon-carbon (C-C) tail of EtOH interacts with the non-polar regions of the isocyanates, contributing to enhanced plasticization [13,14].

Interestingly, previous studies on solvent-stimulated actuation of polyurethanes reported contrasting results, where decreased shape recovery was observed with EtOH compared to water. This discrepancy highlights the significance of specific interactions between the chosen solvent and the polymer chemistry in determining the shape recovery effect [12]. The SMP foam compositions used in these studies were intentionally designed for increased hydrophobicity and reduced water plasticization, as reported by Hasan et al. [15]. The presence of methyl groups in the isocyanate monomers, combined with the ring structure of isophorone diisocyanate (IPDI), inhibits water penetration into the polymer backbone, thereby limiting available isocyanate linkages for water-induced plasticization.

The hypothesis suggests that the unique structure of EtOH, with both polar (OH) and non-polar (C-C tail) regions, allows for significantly increased interactions with the polymer backbone compared to water and DMSO. This molecular flexibility of EtOH enables effective plasticization by forming hydrogen bonds with urethane linkages and interacting with non-polar regions of the polymer [12].

Further investigation is essential to fully understand the mechanisms behind solvent-stimulated SMP foam actuation observed in this study. It is well-known that the relationship between a polymer's structure and its properties is critical in governing its shape memory behavior. By delving into these relationships and mechanisms, researchers can strategically choose solvents and design polymers to improve the performance and functionality of SMPs for various applications that require controlled actuation and shape recovery.

Another fascinating correlation can be understood through the work of Li et al., who developed a system where programmable humidity-responsive actuating behaviors are achieved by incorporating photoprogrammable hygroscopic patterns into SMPs. In their study, they utilized poly(ethylene-co-acrylic acid) (EAA) as a model polymer, and the solvent-processed thin films derived from this material exhibit soft and elastic properties [16]. These films can have their external shapes programmed using a modified shape memory process.

Additionally, Li et al. explored another aspect of their system involving the formation of an Fe^{3+} –carboxylate coordinating network through surface treatments. Under UV light, this network can be spatially dissociated, leading to the creation of transient hygroscopic gradients. These gradients serve as active joints for moisture-driven actuation within the polymer system. This innovative approach opens up new possibilities for developing responsive materials capable of dynamic behaviors based on environmental stimuli.

Exploring further into the mechanical properties of these polymers, it is observed that the resultant samples of EAA exhibit remarkable softness and elasticity at room temperature, as evidenced by the stress–strain curve depicted in Figure 7.5a. These films demonstrate impressive stretchability, capable of reaching 580% strain with a fracture stress of 17.22 MPa. Furthermore, Figure 7.5b illustrates the changes in the storage modulus (G′) and loss tangent (tan δ) of EAA during a heating step. Notably, the value of G′ gradually decreases from 346.43 to 1.22 MPa as the temperature rises from 25°C to 100°C. This significant decrease in G′ upon heating indicates the activation and suppression of EAA chain mobility, which is crucial for achieving thermoresponsive shape memory behavior [16].

The excellent elasticity of EAA at room temperature enables a unique modified shape memory process, illustrated in Figure 7.5c. In this process, a sample is initially elastically deformed by clamping it between two objects at room temperature. Subsequently, the sample, along with the two objects, is heated to a high temperature (T_{high}) and then cooled back to room temperature. Upon separating the objects, the sample retains a temporary shape that aligns closely with the crack between the two objects, demonstrating effective shape fixation (Figure 7.5d). Reheating the sample to T_{high} allows it to revert to its original shape, quantified by evaluating shape fixity ratios (R_fs) and shape recovery ratios (R_rs) obtained by varying T_{high} [16].

The implementability of the proposed shape memory behavior is enhanced by the soft and elastic nature of EAA, contrasting with the rigidity and brittleness of most thermoresponsive SMPs at room temperature. Unlike SMPs that require elevated temperatures for elastic deformation, EAA allows for programming at room temperature, simplifying the process and enabling the creation of temporary shapes with higher intricacy.

Figure 7.5e further demonstrates the elasticity and shape memory behavior of EAA, showcasing its ability to undergo easy stretching and immediate recovery of elastic deformation at room temperature. Leveraging its softness and elasticity, EAA films can be processed into various two-dimensional (2D) kirigami shapes, followed by shape programming steps to transform them into complex three-dimensional (3D) structures, as depicted in Figure 7.5f–h. This innovative approach to shape memory in soft SMPs such as EAA holds promise for further exploration and application in advanced materials science.

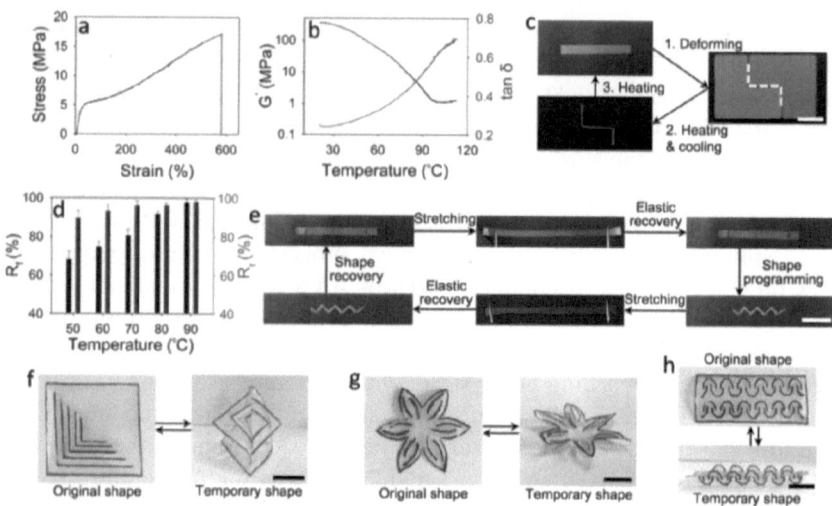

FIGURE 7.5 (a) Stress–strain curve of the prepared EAA film. (b) Changes of the storage modulus (G′) and the loss tangent (tan δ) as a function of temperature. (c) Photos showing the proposed shape memory process: an EAA sample is placed in between two objects to keep it deformed; afterward, the sample and the molds are together heated to a high temperature (T_{high}) and subsequently cooled to room temperature for shape fixation. Lastly, the shape recovery of the sample is triggered by heating to T_{high} again. The white dotted line in the image indicates the position of the sample. (d) R_fs and R_rs obtained in different shape memory cycles with varied T_{high}. (e) Photos showing the room temperature elasticity of an EAA film during a shape memory cycle. (f–h) Shape memory behaviors of three EAA-based kirigami structures. The bars in the images represent 1 cm. Reprinted with permission from [16], copyright reserved American Chemical Society 2022.

Expanding on the mechanical properties and the influence of structure, these aspects can be translated into the moisture-driven shape memory property. Based on the aforementioned studies, we then demonstrate the humidity-driven actuating behaviors of EAA films with tailored 2D shapes and photoprogrammed hygroscopic surfaces. The customized relative humidity (RH)-responsive actuation of three samples is illustrated in Figure 7.6. Each sample's configuration is detailed to show the overall shape (depicted in yellow) and the irradiated regions (highlighted in green) [16].

In the first case (Figure 7.6a), the sample is shaped into a round form and subsequently subjected to light irradiation in four specific regions. As the environmental RH increases, the bending deformations of these irradiated regions toward the non-irradiated side induce the film to curve into a 3D shape.

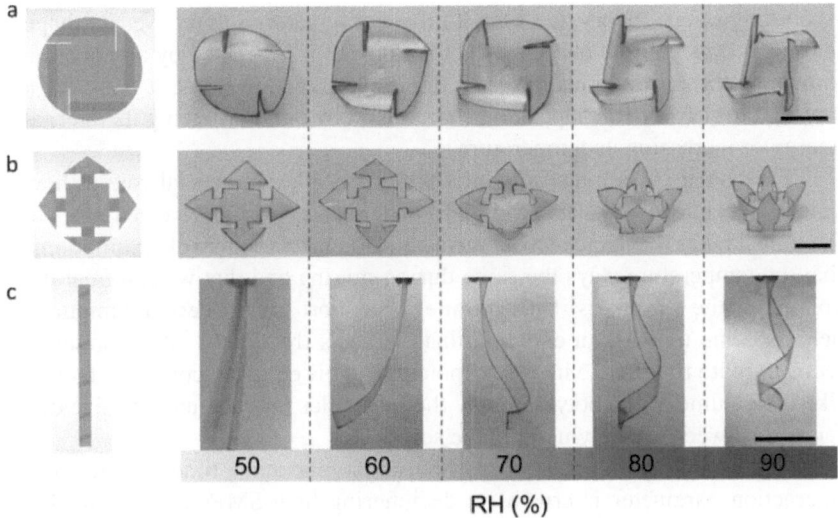

FIGURE 7.6 (a–c) Humidity-responsive actuating behaviors of EAA films with photopatterned hygroscopic surfaces. The yellow regions indicate the geometries of the samples, and the green regions show where the samples are irradiated. The scale bars represent 1 cm. reprinted with permission from [16], copyright reserved American Chemical Society 2022.

This shape gradually reverts back when the RH decreases. Similarly, the second and third samples undergo a similar process: they are initially crafted into designed planar shapes, followed by targeted light irradiation on selected regions. Upon exposure to changing environmental conditions, these samples transform into specific 3D shapes due to humidification and can revert to their original configurations when dried (depicted in Figure 7.6b and 7.6c) [16].

Predicting how solvents affect the recovery of SMPs is quite a puzzle, involving several key factors [17]. When a polymer mixes with a solvent, there's a balance in energy, where the change in free energy for the solvent approaches zero. This means the energy change for the whole system, including the polymer, equals that of the solvent. We also assume the polymer's volume doesn't change during mixing [17].

The decrease in the polymer's energy during mixing is matched with what we call chemo-potential, a measure of how much the system wants to mix. Since energy tends to decrease during mixing, the chemo-potential is always negative. This relationship is represented by a formula involving the number of solvent and polymer molecules, the volume of the polymer, and how the molecules interact. Understanding how SMPs recover their shape also involves some basic principles about how materials relax over time.

According to one theory, the time it takes for a material to recover its shape is linked to its internal energy. This relationship is described by an equation known as the Eyring equation [17]. In simple terms, the time it takes for a material to recover its shape can be shortened by either lowering its internal energy or increasing its temperature.

The change in a material's internal energy plays a crucial role in how quickly it can recover its shape [18]. To understand how this change relates to the time it takes for shape recovery, we need to make a couple of assumptions: that the temperature stays the same during mixing and that we can treat the volume of the solvent as if it's infinite for a short time. These assumptions help us come up with an equation that connects the time it takes for shape recovery with the change in chemo-potential. This equation considers factors like the volume of the polymer, how the molecules interact, and the size difference between the polymer and the solvent.

Understanding the relationship between relaxation time and the FH interaction parameter is crucial in deciphering how SMPs respond to different solvent environments [19]. The FH solution theory provides a mathematical framework for analyzing the thermodynamics of polymer solutions, particularly considering the significant differences in molecular size. The Hildebrand solubility parameter, a numerical estimate of interaction strength, serves as a useful indicator of solubility, especially in polymer materials. When polymers have similar solubility parameters, they tend to interact with each other, leading to phenomena like salvation, miscibility, or swelling [17].

The FH interaction parameter captures the difference in solubility parameters and reflects the interactions between the polymer and the solvent. With a fixed volume ratio between polymer and solvent molecules, relaxation time gradually decreases as the volume fraction of SMP molecules decreases in the solution system. These curves reveal that as the volume fraction of SMP molecules decreases, the mixing chemo-potential initially increases and then decreases. Conversely, as the FH interaction parameter increases, mixing entropy and chemo-potential also increase [17].

An increase in mixing chemo-potential leads to a greater release of energy from the polymer, subsequently decreasing the internal energy of the SMP and indirectly lowering the transition temperature [20,21]. This finding is essential in understanding the SME in SMPs. At elevated temperatures, deformation induced by applied load can be fixed during cooling, storing the work performed as latent strain energy. When the internal energy reaches a critical level, this stored strain energy is released, driving the shape recovery of the SMP.

Finally, the relationship between relaxation time and the volume ratio of polymer to solvent molecules sheds light on how SMPs respond to their environment. In polymer solution theory and relaxation theory, it's understood that internal energy and relaxation time are influenced either by the FH interaction parameter or by the volume dissimilarity between the polymer and solvent molecule [17]. This relationship is derived from the connection between entropy change and volume dissimilarity.

For a real synthetic polymer, there's a statistical distribution of chain lengths, so the volume dissimilarity parameter, denoted as N, represents an average. Imagine each polymer and solvent molecule occupying sites on a lattice, with each site hosting only one molecule [21]. As the volume dissimilarity decreases, the likelihood of a lattice site being occupied by a polymer molecule decreases while the probability of it being occupied by a solvent molecule increases. Consequently, the volume fraction of solvent molecules in the mixture system, occupying lattice sites, increases [17,21].

The decrease in internal energy intensifies as the volume fraction of polymer molecules decreases, leading to a shorter relaxation time [17–21]. This effect is significant across a range of volume dissimilarities, indicating that an increase in the volume ratio between polymers and solvent molecules makes it more challenging to reduce mixing entropy change. Additionally, for a given SMP with the same average volume dissimilarity, the relaxation time decreases as the volume fraction of polymer molecules decreases [17–20].

It's important to note that in systems with strong interactions between monomeric units via hydrogen bonds, the energy of these favorable contacts needs to be considered when inserting a solvent molecule between them during mixing. This necessitates adjustments to parameters like the integral interaction parameter and FH interaction parameter. Despite these considerations, the fundamental understanding remains consistent, highlighting the intricate interplay between the polymer and the solvent molecules in shaping the relaxation behavior of SMPs.

Continuing the discussion recent advancements in biomaterials research have led to the development of cell culture substrates with precisely engineered topographies, revolutionizing the study of cell mechanobiology [22]. These substrates offer researchers unprecedented control over the physical environment in which cells grow, allowing for the exploration of how surface features influence cellular behavior and function. Moreover, these substrates have garnered attention in the field of biomedical device design, where they are employed to enhance the integration of implants with surrounding tissues by promoting cell adhesion and tissue ingrowth [22].

Within this context, SMPs have emerged as a particularly promising material for investigating the impact of surface topography on cell culture dynamics. By utilizing SMPs, researchers can precisely control changes in surface morphology and observe their effects on cell adhesion, proliferation, and differentiation. This approach provides valuable insights into how cells interact with their microenvironment and how these interactions influence tissue development and regeneration [23].

Self-assembly, a fundamental process in both natural and engineered systems, plays a pivotal role in driving the organization of structures at various length scales. While genetic factors dictate the initial blueprint for self-assembly, physical mechanisms ultimately dictate the formation of complex structures. Understanding these mechanisms is crucial for designing biomaterials with tailored properties that mimic the native extracellular matrix and promote tissue regeneration [22–24].

In tissue engineering, the ability to control the shape and structure of organs during their early growth stages is of paramount importance. Techniques such as organ printing, which utilizes computer-aided jet-based three-dimensional tissue generation, hold great promise for fabricating complex tissue constructs with precise control over their geometry and architecture. However, achieving optimal organ shape and structure remains a significant challenge that requires innovative solutions [22].

One such solution lies in the utilization of chemo-responsive SME to create micro/nano-sized surface features on biomaterial substrates. These features, such as wrinkles and protrusion/indentation arrays, provide an effective means of modulating surface morphology to influence cell behavior. By precisely engineering surface topography, researchers can induce specific cellular responses, including changes in cell adhesion, migration, and proliferation. This, in turn, enables the design of biomaterials that better mimic the native cellular microenvironment and promote tissue regeneration [22–24].

Polymers possess unique properties based on their molecular structure, including factors such as crosslinking density and chemical composition. These characteristics directly impact their ability to undergo reversible shape changes in response to external stimuli, such as exposure to solvents. Understanding how solvents interact with specific polymer chemistries and influence polymer chain mobility and conformation is key to developing customized SMPs with desired actuation and recovery properties.

By applying knowledge of structure-property relationships, researchers can optimize SMP formulations to achieve specific actuation behaviors. This involves selecting solvents that effectively modify the polymer backbone without compromising mechanical strength or durability. Additionally, designing polymers with well-defined molecular architectures and crosslinking densities can enhance the efficiency and reliability of shape memory responses.

Ultimately, gaining control over actuation and shape recovery in SMPs through thoughtful polymer design and solvent selection offers promising applications across various industries. These include areas like biomedical devices, textiles, aerospace components, and other technologies where programmable shape change capabilities are valuable. Continued research into these fundamental interactions will expand the potential of SMPs to address diverse practical challenges in innovative and effective ways.

REFERENCES

1. Tang, Z., Deng, G., Cao, P., Gong, J., Yang, J., Yang, Z., ... & Zhang, Y. (2023). Reconfigurable, solvent-processable, NIR-triggerable shape memory cyanate esters for smart molds. *ACS Applied Materials & Interfaces*, *15*(20), 24968–24977.
2. Zhang, F., Wang, L., Geng, Q., Liu, Y., Leng, J., & Smoukov, S. K. (2023). Adjustable volume and loading release of shape memory polymer microcapsules. *International Journal of Smart and Nano Materials*, *14*(1), 77–89.
3. Basak, S., & Bandyopadhyay, A. (2024). Next-gen biomimetic actuators: Bilayer hydrogel evolution in the 21st century and its advancements from a post-2020 perspective. *RSC Appl. Polym.*, 2024, 2, 583–605
4. Basak, S., Angel, J. C. M., & Cavicchi, K. A. (2023). Thermal annealing of high cis-1, 4-polybutadiene/octadecyl acrylate blends as a one-step process for fabricating shape memory polymers. *ACS Applied Polymer Materials*, *5*(7), 4738–4752.
5. Basak, S., & Bandyopadhyay, A. (2024). Toward making polymer chemistry autonomous. *ACS Applied Engineering Materials*. DOI: 10.1021/acsaenm.4c00214
6. Xiao, R., & Huang, W. M. (2020). Heating/solvent responsive shape-memory polymers for implant biomedical devices in minimally invasive surgery: Current status and challenge. *Macromolecular Bioscience*, *20*(8), 2000108.
7. Alexander, S., Xiao, R., & Nguyen, T. D. (2014). Modeling the thermoviscoelastic properties and recovery behavior of shape memory polymer composites. *Journal of Applied Mechanics*, *81*(4), 041003.
8. Nguyen, T. D., Qi, H. J., Castro, F., & Long, K. N. (2008). A thermoviscoelastic model for amorphous shape memory polymers: Incorporating structural and stress relaxation. *Journal of the Mechanics and Physics of Solids*, *56*(9), 2792–2814.
9. Basak, S., & Bandyopadhyay, A. (2022). Two-way semicrystalline shape memory elastomers: Development and current research trends. *Advanced Engineering Materials*, *24*(10), 2200257.
10. Mohan, T. P., George, A. P., & Kanny, K. (2012). Combined effect of isophthalic acid and polyethylene glycol in polyethylene terephthalate polymer on thermal, mechanical, and gas transport properties. *Journal of Applied Polymer Science*, *126*(2), 536–543.
11. Lv, H. B., Liu, Y. J., Zhang, D. X., Leng, J. S., & Du, S. Y. (2008). Solution-responsive shape-memory polymer driven by forming hydrogen bonding. *Advanced Materials Research*, *47*, 258–261.
12. Boyle, A. J., Weems, A. C., Hasan, S. M., Nash, L. D., Monroe, M. B. B., & Maitland, D. J. (2016). Solvent stimulated actuation of polyurethane-based shape memory polymer foams using dimethyl sulfoxide and ethanol. *Smart Materials and Structures*, *25*(7), 075014.
13. Lu, H., Huang, W. M., Fu, Y. Q., & Leng, J. (2014). Quantitative separation of the influence of hydrogen bonding of ethanol/water mixture on the shape recovery behavior of polyurethane shape memory polymer. *Smart Materials and Structures*, *23*(12), 125041.

14. Du, H., & Zhang, J. (2010). Solvent induced shape recovery of shape memory polymer based on chemically cross-linked poly (vinyl alcohol). *Soft Matter*, *6*(14), 3370–3376.
15. Hasan, S. M., Raymond, J. E., Wilson, T. S., Keller, B. K., & Maitland, D. J. (2014). Effects of isophorone diisocyanate on the thermal and mechanical properties of shape-memory polyurethane foams. *Macromolecular Chemistry and Physics*, *215*(24), 2420–2429.
16. Xue, J., Ge, Y., Liu, Z., Liu, Z., Jiang, J., & Li, G. (2022). Photoprogrammable moisture-responsive actuation of a shape memory polymer film. *ACS Applied Materials & Interfaces*, *14*(8), 10836–10843.
17. Lu, H. (2013). State diagram of phase transition temperatures and solvent-induced recovery behavior of shape-memory polymer. *Journal of Applied Polymer Science*, *127*(4), 2896–2904.
18. Yang, Y., & Urban, M. W. (2013). Self-healing polymeric materials. *Chemical Society Reviews*, *42*(17), 7446–7467.
19. Lu, H., Leng, J., & Du, S. (2013). A phenomenological approach for the chemo-responsive shape memory effect in amorphous polymers. *Soft Matter*, *9*(14), 3851–3858.
20. Guo, J., Liu, J., Wang, Z., He, X., Hu, L., Tong, L., & Tang, X. (2017). A thermodynamics viscoelastic constitutive model for shape memory polymers. *Journal of Alloys and Compounds*, *705*, 146–155.
21. Lu, H., & Du, S. (2014). A phenomenological thermodynamic model for the chemo-responsive shape memory effect in polymers based on Flory–Huggins solution theory. *Polymer Chemistry*, *5*(4), 1155–1162.
22. Lu, H., & Huang, W. M. (2015). Chemo-responsive shape-memory polymers for biomedical applications. L'Hocine Yahia (Ed.), In *Shape memory polymers for biomedical applications* (pp. 99–132). Woodhead Publishing.
23. Davis, K. A., Burke, K. A., Mather, P. T., & Henderson, J. H. (2011). Dynamic cell behavior on shape memory polymer substrates. *Biomaterials*, *32*(9), 2285–2293.
24. Jakab, K., Neagu, A., Mironov, V., Markwald, R. R., & Forgacs, G. (2004). Engineering biological structures of prescribed shape using self-assembling multicellular systems. *Proceedings of the National Academy of Sciences*, *101*(9), 2864–2869.

Conclusions and Future Outlook

8

In the realm of biomedicine, precision is key to transforming treatment strategies. This transformation is fueled by the development of Smart Polymeric Materials (SMPs), which can respond to specific signals or triggers in their environment. These materials are incredibly versatile and can be programmed to release drugs with exceptional accuracy, triggered by the presence of certain molecules or conditions in the body [1].

This level of control is particularly promising in fields like oncology and infectious diseases. In cancer treatment, for example, SMPs can target cancer cells specifically, reducing side effects compared to traditional therapies. Similarly, in fighting infections, SMPs can deliver antimicrobial drugs precisely where they're needed, improving treatment effectiveness and reducing the risk of resistance. The ability to fine-tune drug delivery with SMPs represents a significant advancement in medical care. It allows for tailored treatments that meet individual patient needs, improving outcomes and minimizing side effects. As research progresses, integrating SMPs into medical practice could revolutionize how we approach treatment, offering more effective and personalized options for patients.

In cancer treatment, chemotherapy has long been known to be effective against cancer cells, but it's also notorious for causing collateral damage to healthy tissues. This unintended harm leads to a range of unpleasant side effects, such as nausea, fatigue, and hair loss, making the treatment journey particularly challenging for patients. However, the introduction of Smart Polymeric Materials is changing the landscape of cancer therapy [1,2].

Unlike traditional chemotherapy, which affects both cancerous and healthy cells indiscriminately, SMPs offer a more targeted approach. These smart polymers can be meticulously engineered to recognize and selectively deliver therapeutic drugs only to cancer cells, while sparing healthy tissue from harm. By programming SMPs to respond specifically to molecular markers associated with cancer cells, medical researchers are aiming to ensure that the

DOI: 10.1201/9781003593805-8

121

treatment hits its target precisely, minimizing the risk of side effects [1,2]. This targeted chemotherapy strategy holds immense promise for improving patient outcomes and enhancing their quality of life during cancer treatment. With SMPs, the hope is to alleviate the burden of side effects commonly associated with conventional chemotherapy, making the treatment experience more manageable and less distressing for patients [2]. As ongoing research continues to refine and expand the capabilities of SMPs, the potential impact on cancer care is profound, offering new avenues for more effective and patient-friendly treatment options.

In the context of infectious diseases, especially in the battle against drug-resistant organisms, dissolvable responsive SMPs represent a groundbreaking advancement. Drug-resistant bacteria and microorganisms pose a significant threat to public health as they can render conventional antibiotics ineffective. SMPs equipped with solubility-responsive properties can play a pivotal role in combating these resistant pathogens. These polymers can be designed to release antimicrobial agents selectively in the presence of specific microbial markers or environmental conditions associated with infection. This targeted and responsive drug delivery system has the potential to enhance the effectiveness of antimicrobial treatments while minimizing the risk of antimicrobial resistance development. It provides a promising avenue for developing innovative strategies to tackle infectious diseases and overcome the challenges posed by drug-resistant microorganisms. The development of Smart Polymeric Materials (SMPs) represents a paradigm shift in the field of biomedicine. These polymers offer the ability to deliver therapeutic agents with unparalleled precision, responding to specific cues in the environment. In oncology, SMPs enable targeted chemotherapy delivery, reducing the adverse effects of treatment. In infectious diseases, these polymers can selectively release antimicrobial agents, potentially revolutionizing the fight against drug-resistant organisms. The era of precision medicine is upon us, promising more effective and less harmful treatments for a wide range of medical conditions. Tissue designing is another boondock where dissolvable responsive SMPs sparkle splendidly. These versatile materials can act as frameworks for tissue development, progressively changing their shape and properties to mirror the regular extracellular climate [3]. This imaginative methodology encourages further developed tissue recovery, making it conceivable to fix harmed organs, reestablish capability, and even make bio-artificial tissues and organs. The ramifications for patients anticipating organ transfers are significant as dissolvable responsive SMPs could assist with overcoming any issues between organ lack and life-saving medicines [3].

Concerning minimally invasive surgical procedures and medical devices, solvent-responsive shape memory polymers (SMPs) have the potential to introduce a transformative paradigm in the way clinical interventions are conducted [4]. Contemplate a scenario where surgical instruments possess the capability to alter their shape seamlessly within the confines of the human body, thereby facilitating procedures of greater precision through smaller incisions. These "intelligent" instruments stand to enhance surgical outcomes significantly, mitigate patient trauma, and expedite the postoperative recovery process [4].

Furthermore, the development of medical implants crafted from solvent-responsive SMPs represents a substantial stride forward in medical innovation. These implants exhibit an inherent capacity to adapt to the surrounding biological tissue, diminishing the likelihood of complications, elevating patient comfort levels, and extending the overall longevity of the implant itself. Such advancements have the potential to usher in a new era of patient care marked by enhanced surgical techniques and improved implant performance [5,6]. The integration of solvent-responsive SMPs into the field of minimally invasive surgery and medical implants promises to redefine the standards of medical practice. As research and development efforts continue to progress, these materials are poised to contribute significantly to the enhancement of surgical precision, patient outcomes, and the overall quality of healthcare delivery [5,6].

In general, solvent-responsive SMPs have been of growing interest post-2020s. Smoukov et al. recently developed a series of oil-in-water core-shell structure polyurethane (PU) microcapsules with multi-stimuli-responsive properties using the innovative technique of interfacial polymerization. These microcapsules stand out due to their ability to be precisely tuned in terms of surface morphology, providing a high degree of control over their physical attributes, which is a significant advantage in various biomedical applications [7]. Furthermore, these microcapsules exhibit a remarkable shape memory function that sets them apart from conventional capsules and particles. This unique characteristic allows them to revert to their original shape after deformation, making them highly promising for applications such as controlled drug release within the human body. Notably, the microcapsules exhibit a release temperature of 35.4°C, which is lower than typical body temperature, enhancing their suitability for therapeutic use. Moreover, these microcapsules display a distinctive solvent-responsive behavior. When exposed to specific organic solvents, they undergo controlled swelling, ultimately leading to rupture and the release of their encapsulated contents. This property holds significant potential for precisely controlled drug delivery, offering a level of precision and predictability crucial in pharmaceutical applications [7].

While substantial progress has been made in understanding and harnessing the capabilities of these multi-stimuli-responsive microcapsules, it is imperative to acknowledge that there exists an extensive reservoir of untapped potential within this domain [8]. The current study has provided valuable insights into a subset of the response behaviors exhibited by these microcapsules. However, it is crucial to recognize that a myriad of unexplored possibilities and uncharted territories lie beyond the scope of our current investigation [8].

The multi-dimensional nature of these microcapsules suggests that their utility extends far beyond the applications that have been examined thus far. Each facet of their response mechanisms, whether it involves their shape memory functions, solvent-responsive behavior, or other as-yet-undiscovered properties, harbors the potential for transformative advancements across a spectrum of fields. This expansive potential transcends the boundaries of biomedicine and encompasses diverse disciplines such as materials science, nanotechnology, and beyond [9].

Notably, the notion of multi-stimuli-responsiveness hints at a wealth of innovative functionalities that remain concealed, awaiting elucidation. Beyond the stimuli that have been considered in our current study, unexplored triggers or combinations thereof may exist, capable of unlocking hitherto unprecedented capabilities within these microcapsules. Additionally, the synergy arising from the interaction of various stimuli and the resulting emergent behaviors may give rise to groundbreaking solutions, spanning applications from precise drug delivery to the design of advanced materials.

The uncharted terrain of future research and development in this domain is undeniably enticing. It calls for interdisciplinary collaboration, imaginative exploration, and rigorous scientific inquiry to fully actualize the potential of these microcapsules. Delving into the intricacies of their response mechanisms, pioneering innovative synthesis techniques, and tailoring their applications for specific purposes all beckon researchers and innovators to embark on an intellectual journey of immense promise.

In navigating this uncharted terrain, it is imperative to maintain an open-minded and inquisitive approach. Such an approach not only addresses the challenges that lie ahead but also embraces the opportunities presented by a frontier of limitless potential. As we embark on this expedition into the world of multi-stimuli-responsive materials, we anticipate not only the unraveling of groundbreaking discoveries but also the genesis of innovations that stand poised to reshape industries, elevate the standards of healthcare, and confront pressing global challenges. In this light, the full spectrum of response behaviors exhibited by these microcapsules is not just a challenge but an invitation—an invitation to explore, innovate, and ultimately redefine the boundaries of scientific and technological advancement [10].

The authors believe that the integration of 4D printing with solvent responsiveness to target biomedical applications shall be the next scientific disruption. The realm of advanced manufacturing techniques, particularly 4D printing, and associated additive manufacturing methodologies has garnered considerable attention in the pursuit of developing intelligent polymers with intricate architectural features that exhibit responsive behaviors. 4D printing has been widely used in case of thermoresponsive SMPs currently [11–15]; however, its focus on solvent responsive and targeted for biomedical application is still limited owing to the fabrication and the responsiveness challenges.

However, a noteworthy contribution in this context comes from the work of Song et al., who introduced a groundbreaking approach in the creation of shape memory bilayers. These bilayers are composed of polyurethane and a commercially available heat-shrinkable polyethylene, and they are fabricated using gradient 4D printing techniques. This innovative methodology allows for the precise control of the distribution of water-sensitive materials within the bilayer through extrusion-based gradient 3D printing. Consequently, specific and targeted areas within the bilayer can swell differentially, resulting in complex and site-specific shape memory behaviors[16]. The active material developed through this approach demonstrates a dual responsiveness to humidity and temperature stimuli. When exposed to humidity, the polyurethane layer swells, generating a non-uniform strain distribution between the two layers, thereby inducing a bending motion in the material. Subsequently, when the moisture is evaporated, the strain distribution normalizes, leading to the material's recovery to its initial state. This captivating behavior serves as a proof of concept with diverse practical applications [16].

Nonetheless, while we enthusiastically explore the revolutionary potential of solvent-responsive SMPs in the realm of biomedicine, it is imperative that we acknowledge and confront the associated challenges. These challenges must be carefully considered and addressed to ensure the safe and effective utilization of SMPs in biomedical contexts [17,18].

One of the primary challenges revolves around maintaining the mechanical integrity of these materials during shape transitions. As SMPs respond to solvent-induced changes, it is essential to safeguard their structural strength. Striking the delicate balance between flexibility and robustness is an enduring pursuit within the realm of materials science and engineering. Ensuring that the transformative capabilities of SMPs do not compromise their fundamental integrity is paramount to their successful integration into medical applications [18].

Another noteworthy challenge pertains to the time required for shape recovery. In numerous medical scenarios, the expeditious restoration of the original shape is not just desirable but imperative. For instance, in emergency medical devices or situations where timely responses are critical, minimizing the recovery time is of utmost importance. Researchers and engineers are actively engaged in the endeavor to accelerate the recovery process without compromising other essential material properties. This challenge necessitates the exploration of innovative solutions and novel approaches [19].

Furthermore, the synthesis and application of solvent-responsive SMPs in the realm of biomedicine represent a significant leap forward in the trajectory of medical science and healthcare. This convergence of advanced materials science, polymer engineering, and medical technology heralds an era where precision medicine, regenerative therapies, and minimally invasive procedures can deliver unparalleled benefits to patients across the globe [20]. However, it is crucial that we navigate these promising waters with a keen awareness of the challenges at hand, striving for solutions that ensure the safe and effective deployment of SMPs in medical contexts [19–21].

The potential for these materials to enhance therapeutic precision, accelerate tissue regeneration, and revolutionize surgical techniques presents captivating prospects. However, the journey forward is not without its obstacles, and it will require collaboration between researchers, clinicians, and industry partners to overcome these challenges and unlock the full potential of solvent-responsive SMPs in the service of humanity's health and well-being. As we continue to explore and innovate, we stand on the cusp of a medical revolution that promises to reshape healthcare and improve the quality of life for countless individuals around the globe [21].

As a final thought, we want to answer where this trajectory of the development of solvent-responsive SMP shall go. The current landscape of the SMP market is indeed noteworthy, with its size estimated at a substantial USD 392.4 million. What is even more striking is the trajectory it is projected to follow—a robust compound annual growth rate of 21.5% is anticipated from 2021 to 2027, according to reliable sources [22].

This significant growth trajectory can be attributed to several factors that converge to create a fertile ground for the expansion of SMPs. One pivotal driver is the escalating demand for commercialized products that rely on shape morphing capabilities. As industries across the spectrum, from healthcare and aerospace to automotive and consumer electronics, recognize the transformative potential of SMPs, the need for innovative solutions has surged [22]. These polymers possess the unique ability to undergo reversible shape changes upon the application of specific stimuli, making them invaluable in various applications where adaptability and responsiveness are paramount.

Applications are the ultimate goal of all fundamental investigations in SMPs. These materials offer immense potential for innovative design and functionality. The structure model proposed by Hu and Chen highlights SMPs' design capabilities [23], while Xie's research showcases their programmability [24]. Additionally, Ji et al. have explored the diverse shape changes and properties that SMPs can exhibit [25], and Meng and Hu have summarized the various triggering stimuli that can activate these changes

[26]. With such versatility, the application potential for SMPs appears nearly limitless, and their use in various fields is expected to continue growing in the coming years.

Biomedical applications have been a major focus in SMP research over the past decade and will likely remain a key area. The future may bring mature technologies in tissue engineering, tissue repair, minimally invasive surgery, controllable drug delivery, and biodegradability and biocompatibility of SMPs. Another area of current interest is textiles, where shape memory fibers have been developed for applications in sportswear, intimate apparel, and industrial uses. Collaborations between institutions like the Hong Kong Polytechnic University and international companies have produced prototypes, indicating that SMPs could achieve significant commercial success in the next five years [26].

Beyond medicine and textiles, SMP applications are expanding into new fields. The aircraft and space industries, as well as the military, are promising areas due to the unique properties of SMPs, such as light weight, large volume change, flexibility, and controlled, gradual recovery processes. This controlled recovery is crucial for avoiding vibrations that could damage systems in space. Surface and thin film applications should also see increased attention, leveraging the small recovery forces typical of SMPs. Emerging applications include energy harvesting from solar (light-responsive SMPs) and chemical sources (chemical-responsive SMPs) and two-way SMPs for cyclical deformation, similar to artificial muscles found in shape memory alloys (SMAs). These areas hold high value and social importance, potentially drawing significant future research efforts.

The research and development efforts aimed at crafting novel SMPs are poised to be a game-changer within the current landscape [14,27]. These endeavors hold the promise of not merely expanding the existing boundaries but of fundamentally reshaping the way we perceive and utilize shape memory materials. This transformative shift is expected to have far-reaching implications, impacting industries and applications that range from medical devices and robotics to aerospace engineering and beyond [14,27–30].

The projected growth and evolution of the SMP market symbolize a dynamic convergence of scientific innovation, engineering prowess, and industrial demand. As the journey unfolds, it is poised to usher in a new era marked by unprecedented advancements in materials science and engineering [14,27–31]. These developments are expected to revolutionize industries and bring forth novel solutions that were once deemed unattainable. Thus, the future of solvent-responsive SMPs appears exceptionally promising, with opportunities for groundbreaking breakthroughs and transformative applications on the horizon.

REFERENCES

1. Brentnall, A. R., Harkness, E. F., Astley, S. M., Donnelly, L. S., Stavrinos, P., Sampson, S., ... & Evans, D. G. R. (2015). Mammographic density adds accuracy to both the Tyrer-Cuzick and Gail breast cancer risk models in a prospective UK screening cohort. *Breast Cancer Research, 17*, 1–10.
2. Ting, A. H., McGarvey, K. M., & Baylin, S. B. (2006). The cancer epigenome—components and functional correlates. *Genes & Development, 20*(23), 3215–3231.
3. Hasan, S. M., Nash, L. D., & Maitland, D. J. (2016). Porous shape memory polymers: Design and applications. *Journal of Polymer Science Part B: Polymer Physics, 54*(14), 1300–1318.
4. Wang, C. C., Huang, W. M., Ding, Z., Zhao, Y., & Purnawali, H. (2012). Cooling-/water-responsive shape memory hybrids. *Composites Science and Technology, 72*(10), 1178–1182.
5. Wang, X. (2022). A coupling model for the cooperative actuation mechanism of thermochemically responsive shape memory polymers. *Smart Materials and Structures, 31*(12), 125001.
6. Lu, H., & Huang, W. M. (2015). Chemo-responsive shape-memory polymers for biomedical applications. In *Shape memory polymers for biomedical applications* (pp. 99–132). Woodhead Publishing.
7. Zhang, F., Wang, L., Geng, Q., Liu, Y., Leng, J., & Smoukov, S. K. (2023). Adjustable volume and loading release of shape memory polymer microcapsules. *International Journal of Smart and Nano Materials, 14*(1), 77–89.
8. Wang, K., Jia, Y. G., Zhao, C., & Zhu, X. X. (2019). Multiple and two-way reversible shape memory polymers: Design strategies and applications. *Progress in Materials Science, 105*, 100572.
9. Wang, Y., Cui, H., Esworthy, T., Mei, D., Wang, Y., & Zhang, L. G. (2022). Emerging 4D printing strategies for next-generation tissue regeneration and medical devices. *Advanced Materials, 34*(20), 2109198.
10. Yan, C., Feng, X., Wick, C., Peters, A., & Li, G. (2021). Machine learning assisted discovery of new thermoset shape memory polymers based on a small training dataset. *Polymer, 214*, 123351.
11. Khalid, M. Y., Arif, Z. U., Noroozi, R., Zolfagharian, A., & Bodaghi, M. (2022). 4D printing of shape memory polymer composites: A review on fabrication techniques, applications, and future perspectives. *Journal of Manufacturing Processes, 81*, 759–797.
12. Spiegel, C. A., Hackner, M., Bothe, V. P., Spatz, J. P., & Blasco, E. (2022). 4D printing of shape memory polymers: From macro to micro. *Advanced Functional Materials, 32*(51), 2110580.
13. Zhang, W., Wang, H., Wang, H., Chan, J. Y. E., Liu, H., Zhang, B., ... & Yang, J. K. (2021). Structural multi-colour invisible inks with submicron 4D printing of shape memory polymers. *Nature Communications, 12*(1), 112.
14. Subash, A., & Kandasubramanian, B. (2020). 4D printing of shape memory polymers. *European Polymer Journal, 134*, 109771.
15. Zhang, C., Cai, D., Liao, P., Su, J. W., Deng, H., Vardhanabhuti, B., ... & Lin, J. (2021). 4D Printing of shape-memory polymeric scaffolds for adaptive biomedical implantation. *Acta Biomaterialia, 122*, 101–110.

16. Song, Z., Ren, L., Zhao, C., Liu, H., Yu, Z., Liu, Q., & Ren, L. (2020). Biomimetic nonuniform, dual-stimuli self-morphing enabled by gradient four-dimensional printing. *ACS Applied Materials & Interfaces, 12*(5), 6351–6361.

17. Jian, B., Li, H., He, X., Wang, R., Yang, H. Y., & Ge, Q. (2023). Two-photon polymerization-based 4D printing and its applications. *International Journal of Extreme Manufacturing*.

18. Basak, S. (2023). *Structure-property relationships of high CIS 1,4 polybutadiene based shape memory polymers* [Doctoral dissertation, University of Akron]. OhioLINK Electronic Theses and Dissertations Center. https://rave.ohiolink.edu/etdc/view?acc_num=akron169442793626196

19. Pielichowska, K., & Blazewicz, S. (2010). Bioactive polymer/hydroxyapatite (nano) composites for bone tissue regeneration. In *Biopolymers: Lignin, proteins, bioactive nanocomposites* (pp. 97–207).

20. Fu, Y. Q., Huang, W. M., Luo, J. K., & Lu, H. (2015). Polyurethane shape-memory polymers for biomedical applications. In *Shape memory polymers for biomedical applications* (pp. 167–195). Woodhead Publishing.

21. Huang, W. M. (2010). Thermo-moisture responsive polyurethane shape memory polymer for biomedical devices. *The Open Medical Devices Journal, 2*(1).

22. Basak, S., & Bandyopadhyay, A. (2021). Solvent responsive shape memory polymers-evolution, current status, and future outlook. *Macromolecular Chemistry and Physics, 222*(19), 2100195.

23. Hu, J., & Chen, S. (2010). A review of actively moving polymers in textile applications. *Journal of Materials Chemistry, 20*(17), 3346–3355.

24. Xie, T. (2011). Recent advances in polymer shape memory. *Polymer, 52*(22), 4985–5000.

25. Ji, F. L., Hu, J. L., Li, T. C., & Wong, Y. W. (2007). Morphology and shape memory effect of segmented polyurethanes. Part I: With crystalline reversible phase. *Polymer, 48*(17), 5133–5145.

26. Hu, J., Zhu, Y., Huang, H., & Lu, J. (2012). Recent advances in shape–memory polymers: Structure, mechanism, functionality, modeling and applications. *Progress in Polymer Science, 37*(12), 1720–1763.

27. Basak, S. (2021). Redesigning the modern applied medical sciences and engineering with shape memory polymers. *Advanced Composites and Hybrid Materials, 4*, 223–234.

28. Basak, S., Dasgupta, P., & Bandyopadhyay, A. (2023). One-way shape memory polyesters-evolution, growth, developments, and current trends. *Polymer-Plastics Technology and Materials, 62*(17), 2286–2317.

29. Basak, S., & Bandyopadhyay, A. (2024). Next-gen biomimetic actuators: Bilayer hydrogel evolution in the 21st century and its advancements from a post-2020 perspective. *RSC Applied Polymers*.

30. Sun, L., Wang, T. X., Chen, H. M., Salvekar, A. V., Naveen, B. S., Xu, Q., ... & Huang, W. M. (2019). A brief review of the shape memory phenomena in polymers and their typical sensor applications. *Polymers, 11*(6), 1049.

31. Lendlein, A., Behl, M., Hiebl, B., & Wischke, C. (2010). Shape-memory polymers as a technology platform for biomedical applications. *Expert Review of Medical Devices, 7*(3), 357–379.

Index